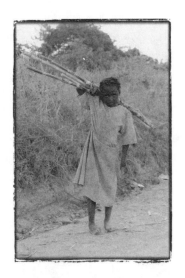

The aWAKE Project

Uniting Against the African AIDS Crisis

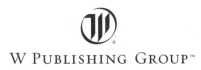

W PUBLISHING GROUP™

www.wpublishinggroup.com

A Division of Thomas Nelson, Inc.
www.ThomasNelson.com

The aWAKE Project: Uniting Against the African AIDS Crisis

Copyright © 2002 by W. Publishing Group

Published by W. Publishing Group, a Thomas Nelson Company,
P.O. Box 141000, Nashville, Tennessee 37214

Compiled by: Jenny Eaton and Kate Etue

Cover Design: Four5One Design, Dublin, Ireland

Cover Photo: Bono

Page Design: Nelson Design Group, Nashville, Tennessee

Title page photo courtesy of Pam Kidd.

The statistics provided in this book may no longer be accurate, as they change daily.
Please visit www.unaids.com for up-to-date information.

The perspective, beliefs, and views of individual contributors do not necessarily
reflect those of Thomas Nelson, Inc. or W Publishing Group.

Library of Congress Cataloging-in-Publication Data

The awake project : uniting against the global AIDS pandemic.
   p. cm.
ISBN 0-8499-4409-0
1. AIDS (Disease)—Africa. 2. AIDS (Disease)
RA643.86.A35 A95 2002
362.1'969792'0096—dc21   2002012158

Printed and bound in the United States of America

02 03 04 05 06 - 5 4 3 2 1

Do this because you know the time;
It is the hour now for you to aWAKE from sleep,
For our salvation is nearer than when we first believed.

—ROMANS 13:11

CONTENTS

Part I

Awareness

CONTENTS

Part II

Knowledge

CONTENTS

Part III

Engagement

CONTENTS

LETTER FROM THE EDITORS

Since the first case was reported in 1981, the HIV/AIDS virus has grown to epic proportions. The death toll has multiplied in America to more than a half million. Some estimates show that every hour two young persons contract the HIV virus. Our generation has lived through the eras of discovery, growth, crisis, and complacency. Even today, HIV/AIDS still lacks a cure, and it continues to struggle for research dollars to move forward with vaccines.

While the HIV/AIDS issue in America continues to be a threat to our nation, the virus in Africa and other regions has become a pandemic. In Africa, thirty-four million people have been infected with HIV; thirteen million are orphans. Every minute two people contract the HIV virus; and 90 percent of those people are children. The number one mode of transmission is not through homosexual activity but from mother to infant. This is indeed the "new plague" of our times. Yet, a Barna Research poll shows that evangelical Christians are the least likely group to help AIDS victims in Africa—less than 3 percent said they would financially help a Christian organization minister to an AIDS orphan.

The aWAKE Project is the first book of its kind to target a general audience: AIDS: Working toward Awareness, Knowledge, and Engagement. We want the citizens of the world to *wake up* to this devastating disease that is killing our brothers and sisters across the nations. Upon awareness, we mourn the loss of these fellow human beings in a global *wake*, or funeral, for life itself. And, finally, we hope a *wake* of emotional and intellectual response follows worldwide by spreading knowledge for the sake of action.

In this book musicians, politicians, actors, athletes, writers, speakers, activists, experts, religious, and non-religious unite with

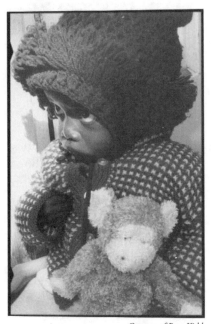

Courtesy of Pam Kidd

one voice to speak to their realization, understanding, and experience of the pandemic in their own lives. It is our hope that you will hear the voices of those you know and respect as they speak wisdom from their corner of the world.

But, how can you get involved? We have incorporated a number of organizations in the back of the book for you to join. Our Engagement section offers different levels of involvement from writing your senator to mobilizing other groups. Be ambassadors for life to a dying continent.

Our many thanks to those who have given graciously to create this book: All contributors generously donated their pieces for no fee—for that we wish to offer our appreciation.

—*Jenny Eaton and Kate Etue, Editors*

The Publisher would like to remind the reader that it neither endorses nor necessarily agrees with positions that contributors may (or may not) represent. Each contributor has generously offered his or her article because s/he realizes the crisis situation of AIDS in the world and the need for urgency. We believe that even though we (Publisher, Contributors, and Organizations) may not agree on all aspects relating to the crisis, we all need to work together to defeat AIDS with God's help. Thank you.

FOREWORD

HIV/AIDS: The Plague of Our Time

Melvin L. Cheatham, M.D.

Acquired Immunodeficiency Syndrome (AIDS), is a deadly disease caused by a retrovirus called HIV. AIDS was unknown until the first cases were identified in 1981. Today, it is spreading rampant around the world, causing untold suffering and millions of deaths. It is "The Plague" of our time.

The word *plague* conjures up memories from the Bible of the great afflictions brought by God upon the people of Egypt. Over the course of the past millennium, our world experienced the great Bubonic plague, referred to as "The Black Death." This affliction was caused by the Yersinia pestis bacterium, and it was carried by fleas in the fur of rats. Millions upon millions of people died of this terrible disease as it swept across Europe and North Africa, destroying not only people's lives but disrupting entire societies.

History is replete with accounts of terrible pandemics that have taken deadly tolls. During the 1800s Europe and North America suffered four devastating pandemics of cholera. America had its own plague as the great influenza pandemic of 1918-19 swept across the country.

In the last twenty-five years, new viral diseases have appeared, and it has been hypothesized they have come from the darkest forests and the densest jungles of Central Africa. At a time when medical science believed we stood upon the threshold of defeating infectious diseases, people have died terrible, unexplainable deaths.

Because of these great pandemics, societies have been devastated, leaving terrorism, sin and turmoil to emerge from their shreds. In the moral vacuum left in the wake of disease, the forces of evil have often reared their ugly heads. Sin and social disruption have repeatedly been the survivors of the chaos these plagues and pandemics have wrought.

During the final years of the twentieth century, something else started to silently erode away the very foundation of society. The sexual revolution caused a rapid change in what was considered socially and spiritually acceptable for people to think and to do. The world seemed to rapidly become smaller and smaller. Sexually transmitted diseases became rampant as heterosexual behavior with multiple partners, relationships between people of the same sex, and widespread intravenous drug use with shared needles increased.

These radical changes in human behavior also brought a great price: loss of health and human life. One such example appeared in the Fall of 1980. Dr. Michael Gottlieb, a physician in San Francisco, was asked to see a thirty-three year old homosexual patient with an unusual respiratory infection. In the months that followed, Dr. Gottlieb encountered several other patients with this same unusual condition and eventually reported it as a new disease syndrome.

At first AIDS was thought to be a disease only infecting homosexuals, but before long it became terrifyingly obvious that HIV/AIDS is a potential threat to everyone: man, woman, or child. Many millions of people are now infected, and many millions more have already died. Experts tell us we have only seen the tip of this iceberg, and yet many people continue to turn away from it, denying it is even there.

As you read the pages that follow in *The aWAKE Project*, you will find it addresses the burning question looming before us today: *What are we going to do about HIV/AIDS?* The contibutors to this project are people who have chosen not to "turn and look the other way," as the priest and the Levite did in Jesus' story of the Good Samaritan.

May God speak to you as you read this very important book and lead you to find your place in the battle to defeat HIV/AIDS.

Written for The aWAKE Project.
Copyright © 2002 by Melvin L. Cheatham.

PREFACE

Awaken

His Majesty King Mswati III
King of Swaziland

The theme of "awake" to the HIV/AIDS crisis is an interesting juxtaposition of words. *Awaken* is the process of rousing from sleep. Yet to awaken the world to the crisis of the HIV/AIDS pandemic, thousands of African men, women, and children are slipping into their final resting place.

The dire statistics, the pictures, the stories of personal human suffering seem to have only desensitized many people on our planet to the quiet suffering of the African people. The African people stand together with many of the world's leaders, the medical community, and our friends to fight this disease but it just keeps coming—a soulless killer who never rests in the efficient task of invading the blood of our people.

Throughout its history, Africa has suffered from every natural disaster imaginable. HIV/AIDS is the worst. Malaria may kill more, but its victims have hope of surviving if diagnosed in time. HIV/AIDS has killed less, but it has no cure. And at its inception decades ago, it wisely masked itself as a taboo social disease. Today in its maturity, HIV/AIDS kills during birth, in hospitals, and in families.

Just as the disease has matured, so must we. African leaders and leaders throughout the world must treat all those afflicted with compassion, especially the orphans. We must do our part to remove the social stigma of the disease so that no one fears testing, treatment, and education. In Swaziland, we are doing our part with limited resources, and with the help of the entertainment industry we are working to raise awareness among the world's young people through the release of a compact disc entitled *Songs for Life.*

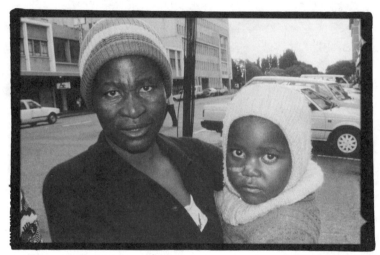

Courtesy of Pam Kidd

In the highlands of my small African country, rich with natural resources and steeped in history, I watch the countless funeral processions and the growing number of freshly dug graves with deep sadness. When I look into the melancholy eyes of the children who have been left behind, I am frustrated by the knowledge that help exists to stop this plague. HIV/AIDS is such a large problem, yet the Kingdom of Swaziland is such a small country. The world needs a victory in the war against HIV/AIDS and Swaziland, as a small country with a modern infrastructure is the ideal place to win the first battle.

Over the past year the world has awoken to the terror and dangers of terrorism. Terrorism will be defeated by the sheer will of decent people who want to live in peace. The HIV/AIDS pandemic is an equal threat to world peace and stability. Over eight thousand people succumb to AIDS each day, six thousand are Africans, and the numbers are growing. Left untreated—or even worse—partially treated, the disease will learn to resist the latest drugs. More will perish, and more children will spend their formative years as orphans outside of the traditional family unit, where values, respect for human dignity, and morals are instilled. Africans have awoken to the threat of HIV/AIDS to our very existence.

Written for The aWAKE Project.

Copyright © 2002 by His Majesty King Mswati III.

INTRODUCTION

Indifferent Christians and the African Crisis

Tony Campolo

I need not go into the agony that Africa is enduring under the impact of the AIDS epidemic. I wish you could see what I saw with my own eyes as I visited South Africa and Zimbabwe. The suffering I witnessed led me to get together the resources to start a program for the orphans of those who have died from AIDS. You meet them almost everywhere you go in those countries. Many of these children have AIDS themselves. Our program is designed to provide them with some loving care and sustenance. No child should be abandoned to the streets, covered with the body sores that accompany AIDS. No child should die alone without knowing that he or she is loved.

The social impact of AIDS is horrendous. In two of the schools I visited, there was a shortage of teachers because several of those who had held teaching positions had been victimized by the disease and were gone. I learned that schools throughout Africa are enduring this same loss of crucial personnel. The very people that Africa needs to emerge out of economic privation are being liquidated by this dreaded disease.

I believe that too often the Christian response to the AIDS epidemic has been abominable. In many instances there is a tendency to write off those who are suffering from AIDS on the grounds that this disease is some kind of punishment from God meted out to those who have been sexually promiscuous. The logic behind such a conclusion is beyond my comprehension. Consider the fact that a huge number of those who are HIV positive are women who have been infected, not because of any immoral behavior on their part, but because their husbands gave them the disease. Are they to be condemned and ignored because of what their husbands have done? And what about the children who are infected? Children constitute a significant proportion of those who are facing the possibility of AIDS-related death through no fault of their own.

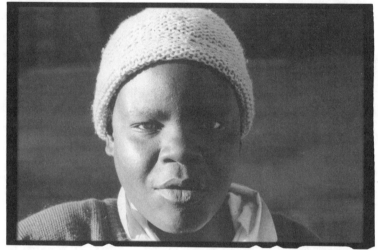

Courtesy of Pam Kidd

The church must recognize that AIDS very much parallels the disease of leprosy that we read about in the New Testament. In Biblical times, those who had leprosy were deemed spiritually unclean, and others would not get near them or touch them for fear of contamination that would be both physically harmful and spiritually defiling. Leprosy was seen to have a spiritual dimension to it and those who had the disease were looked upon as being especially cursed by God. Given those realities about people who had leprosy back then, it is easy to understand why comparisons can be made to those who are infected by AIDS in our contemporary world.

It is important for us to note that Jesus had a special spot in his heart for the lepers. He embraced them. He touched them. He reached out to them in love. All of this was contrary to the legalistic pietism of religious leaders in his day. Jesus' condemnation of such religionists was harsh. He always reached out to the lepers to make them whole, in spite of the fact that touching them would render him ceremoniously unclean to the custodians of the temple religion.

The Jesus who we find in Scripture calls upon us to look for him in the eyes of the poor and the oppressed. He tells us in Matthew 25 that what we do "to the least of them" we do to him. The Christ of Scripture refuses to be an abstraction in the sky. Instead, he chooses to be incarnated in the last, the least, and the lost of this world. I contend that he is especially present in those who suffer from AIDS. Sacramentally, the resurrected Jesus waits to be loved in each of them. Mother Teresa once said, "Whenever I look into the eyes of someone dying of AIDS, I have an eerie awareness that Jesus is staring back at me." Indeed, that is the case. No one can say that he or she loves Jesus without embracing Jesus in those who have this torturous disease.

The indifference on the part of Christians and on the part of the nation in general to those in Africa suffering from AIDS, may reveal a latent racism. There is often an unspoken feeling that since these victims of AIDS are usually black people, those of us who are white might just as well look the other way. You can almost sense that there are those who are inwardly saying, "If millions of them die off, will it not relieve the hunger problem in Africa? Will it not eliminate an large proportion of an undesirable race?" I doubt if we will hear those words out loud, but I have heard statements that imply the same thing, and I am horrified! In Christ there is neither Jew nor Greek; bond nor free; Scythian nor barbarian; male nor female. Anyone who allows racist tendencies to go unchallenged in his or her personality is not living like a Christian. The Scriptures make it clear that anyone who says he or she loves God, and does not love the brother or sister who is a neighbor, is a liar. People suffering from AIDS in Africa *are* our brothers and sisters.

Those of us who are in the church must use what moral

authority we have to speak against those political and economic structures that the Bible refers to as the "principalities and powers" that rule our age. We must raise our voice against those pharmaceutical corporations that overprice the cocktail drugs that could slow down the effects of the HIV virus in those who are infected. We must call the corporate community to account for their apparent tendency to put profits far above people.

We must also speak out against a government that spends trillions of dollars to build up a military machine, but provides only a pittance to deal with the AIDS crisis that is destroying Africa. As we wage war on terrorism, we must be aware that terrorism cannot be eliminated until we deal with the economic imbalances and the social injustices that breed terrorism. When we Americans do so little to help the poor victims of AIDS in Africa, an anger is stirred up that can lead people who are diseased and oppressed to strike at us with vengeance. We do not get rid of malaria by killing mosquitoes. Instead, we must destroy the swamps in which the mosquitoes breed. So it is that we will not get rid of terrorism by killing individual terrorists. In the end, we must get rid of the conditions that breed terrorists. We must attack the poverty and the oppression that nurtures such extremism. Enlightened self-interest should lead us to assume that unless we, who live in the richest nation on the face of the earth, respond to the AIDS crisis in Africa, there will be dire consequences.

But, in the end, we who call ourselves followers of Jesus have a higher calling than our own self-interest. If Christ is a reality in our lives, then our hearts will be broken by the things that break the heart of Jesus. There can be no doubt that the heart of our Lord is broken by what is happening in Africa, even now. If nothing else, our hearts should burn within us as we face the fact that thirteen million children in Africa have been orphaned because of AIDS, and that for each of them Jesus sheds His tears.

On Judgment Day, we will not be asked theological questions. Instead, we will be asked, as it says in Matthew 25, how we responded to those who were poor, diseased, downhearted, and alone. Jesus will ask us on that day if we reached out to the stranger

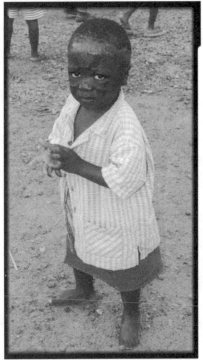

Courtesy of Pam Kidd

in need with loving care and if we treated the sick with true compassion. It is not that theological convictions are unimportant, but rather that true commitment to the beliefs we espouse will be manifested in compassionate action on behalf of those who are writhing in the agonies of AIDS, even now.

Let us remember the chorus of an old gospel hymn that goes:

> *Rescue the perishing,*
> *Care for the dying,*
> *Jesus is merciful,*
> *Jesus will save.*

Written for The aWAKE Project,
Copyright © 2002 by Tony Campolo.

PART ONE

Awareness

EDWARD THOMPSON

Poet, 8 years old

AIDS, My Friend, AIDS

AIDS, my friend, AIDS
Is very dangerous.
AIDS, my friend, AIDS
Is very dangerous.

Look how naked
The world has become—
Empty houses all around,
Children without parents
Crying day and night
But with no answer.

AIDS, my friend, AIDS
Is very dangerous.

People with good papers
Have gone completely.
Please teachers,
Government officials,
Church clergies,
Teach the nation about AIDS.

AIDS, my friend, AIDS
Is very dangerous.

Reprinted by permission of World Vision.

JOHANNA MCGEARY

Journalist

Death Stalks A Continent

In the dry timber of African societies, AIDS was a spark. The conflagration it set off continues to kill millions. Here's why.

Imagine your life this way.

You get up in the morning and breakfast with your three kids. One is already doomed to die in infancy. Your husband works 200 miles away, comes home twice a year and sleeps around in between. You risk your life in every act of sexual intercourse. You go to work past a house where a teenager lives alone tending young siblings without any source of income. At another house, the wife was branded a whore when she asked her husband to use a condom, beaten silly and thrown into the streets. Over there lies a man desperately sick without access to a doctor or clinic or medicine or food or blankets or even a kind word. At work you eat with colleagues, and every third one is already fatally ill. You whisper about a friend who admitted she had the plague and whose neighbors stoned her to death. Your leisure is occupied by the funerals you attend every Saturday. You go to bed fearing adults your age will not live into their 40s. You and your neighbors and your political and popular leaders act as if nothing is happening.

Across the southern quadrant of Africa, this nightmare is real. The word not spoken is AIDS, and here at ground zero of humanity's deadliest cataclysm, the ultimate tragedy is that so many people don't know—or don't want to know—what is happening.

As the HIV virus sweeps mercilessly through these lands—the fiercest trial Africa has yet endured—a few try to address the terrible depredation. The rest of society looks away. Flesh and muscle melt from the bones of the sick in packed hospital wards and lonely bush kraals. Corpses stack up in morgues until those on top crush the identity from the faces underneath. Raw earth mounds scar the landscape, grave after grave without name or number. Bereft children grieve for parents lost in their prime, for siblings scattered to the winds.

The victims don't cry out. Doctors and obituaries do not give the killer its name. Families recoil in shame. Leaders shirk responsibility. The stubborn silence heralds victory for the disease: denial cannot keep the virus at bay.

The developed world is largely silent too. AIDS in Africa has never commanded the full-bore response the West has brought to other, sometimes lesser, travails. We pay sporadic attention, turning on the spotlight when an international conference occurs, then turning it off. Good-hearted donors donate; governments acknowledge that more needs to be done. But think how different the effort would be if what is happening here were happening in the West.

By now you've seen pictures of the sick, the dead, the orphans. You've heard appalling numbers: the number of new infections, the number of the dead, the number who are sick without care, the number walking around already fated to die.

But to comprehend the full horror AIDS has visited on Africa, listen to the woman we have dubbed Laetitia Hambahlane in Durban or the boy Tsepho Phale in Francistown or the woman who calls herself Thandiwe in Bulawayo or Louis Chikoka, a long-distance trucker. You begin to understand how AIDS has struck Africa—with a biblical virulence that will claim tens of millions of lives—when you hear about shame and stigma and ignorance and poverty and sexual violence and migrant labor and promiscuity and political

5

paralysis and the terrible silence that surrounds all this dying. It is a measure of the silence that some asked us not to print their real names to protect their privacy.

Theirs is a story about what happens when a disease leaps the confines of medicine to invade the body politic, infecting not just individuals but an entire society. As AIDS migrated to man in Africa, it mutated into a complex plague with confounding social, economic and political mechanics that locked together to accelerate the virus' progress. The region's social dynamics colluded to spread the disease and help block effective intervention.

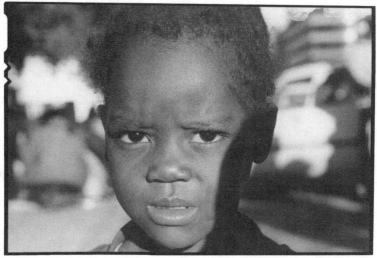

Courtesy of Pam Kidd

We have come to three countries abutting one another at the bottom of Africa—Botswana, South Africa, Zimbabwe—the heart of the heart of the epidemic. For nearly a decade, these nations suffered a hidden invasion of infection that concealed the dimension of the coming calamity. Now the omnipresent dying reveals the shocking scale of the devastation.

AIDS in Africa bears little resemblance to the American epidemic, limited to specific high-risk groups and brought under control through intensive education, vigorous political action and expensive drug therapy. Here the disease has bred a Darwinian perversion. Society's fittest, not its frailest, are the ones who die—adults spirited away, leaving the old and the children behind. You cannot define risk groups: everyone who is sexually active is at risk. Babies too, unwittingly infected by mothers. Barely a single family remains untouched. Most do not know how or when they caught the virus, many never know they have it, many who do know don't tell anyone as they lie dying. Africa can provide no treatment for those with AIDS.

They will all die, of tuberculosis, pneumonia, meningitis, diarrhea, whatever overcomes their ruined immune systems first. And the statistics, grim as they are, may be too low. There is no broad-scale AIDS testing: infection rates are calculated mainly from the presence of HIV in pregnant women. Death certificates in these countries do not record AIDS as the cause. "Whatever stats we have are not reliable," warns Mary Crewe of the University of Pretoria's Center for the Study of AIDS. "Everybody's guessing." . . .

The Outcast

To acknowledge AIDS in yourself is to be branded as monstrous. Laetitia Hambahlane (not her real name) is 51 and sick with AIDS. So is her brother. She admits it; he doesn't. In her mother's broken-down house in the mean streets of Umlazi township, though, Laetitia's mother hovers over her son, nursing him, protecting him, resolutely denying he has anything but TB, though his sister claims the sure symptoms of AIDS mark him. Laetitia is the outcast, first from her family, then from her society.

For years Laetitia worked as a domestic servant in Durban and dutifully sent all her wages home to her mother. She fell in love a number of times and bore four children. "I loved that last man," she recalls. "After he left, I had no one, no sex." That was 1992, but Laetitia already had HIV.

She fell sick in 1996, and her employers sent her to a private doctor who couldn't diagnose an illness. He tested her blood and found she was HIV positive. "I wish I'd died right then," she says, as tears spill down her sunken cheeks. "I asked the doctor, 'Have you got medicine?' He said no. I said, 'Can't you keep me alive?'" The doctor could do nothing and sent her away. "I couldn't face the word," she says. "I couldn't sleep at night. I sat on my bed, thinking, praying. I did not see anyone day or night. I ask God, Why?"

Laetitia's employers fired her without asking her exact diagnosis. For weeks she could not muster the courage to tell anyone. Then she told her children, and they were ashamed and frightened. Then, harder still, she told her mother. Her mother raged about the loss of money if Laetitia could not work again. She was so angry she ordered Laetitia out of the house. When her daughter wouldn't leave, the mother threatened to sell the house to get rid of her daughter. Then she walled off her daughter's room with plywood partitions, leaving the daughter a pariah, alone in a cramped, dark space without windows and only a flimsy door opening into the alley. Laetitia must earn the pennies to feed herself and her children by peddling beer, cigarettes and candy from a shopping cart in her room, when people are brave enough to stop by her door. "Sometimes they buy, sometimes not," she says. "That is how I'm surviving."

Her mother will not talk to her. "If you are not even accepted by your own family," says Magwazi, the volunteer home-care giver from Durban's Sinoziso project who visits Laetitia, "then others will not accept you." When Laetitia ventures outdoors, neighbors snub her, tough boys snatch her purse, children taunt her. Her own kids are tired of the sickness and don't like to help her anymore. "When I can't get up, they don't bring me food," she laments. One day local youths barged into her room, cursed her as a witch and a whore and beat her. When she told the police, the youths returned, threatening to burn down the house.

But it is her mother's rejection that wounds Laetitia most. "She is hiding it about my brother," she cries. "Why will she do nothing for me?" Her hands pick restlessly at the quilt covering her paper-thin frame. "I know my mother will not bury me properly. I know she will not take care of my kids when I am gone."

Jabulani Syabusi would use his real name, but he needs to protect his brother. He teaches school in a red, dusty district of KwaZulu-Natal. People here know the disease is all around them, but no one speaks of it. He eyes the scattered huts that make up his little settlement on an arid bluff. "We can count 20 who died just here as far as we can see. I personally don't remember any family that told it was AIDS," he says. "They hide it if they do know."

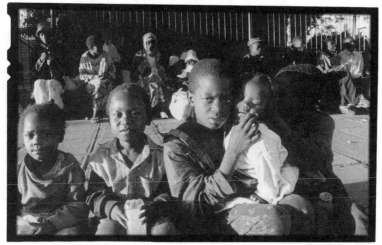

Courtesy of Pam Kidd

Syabusi's own family is no different. His younger brother is also a teacher who has just come home from Durban too sick to work anymore. He says he has tuberculosis, but after six months the tablets he is taking have done nothing to cure him. Syabusi's wife Nomsange, a nurse, is concerned that her 36-year-old brother-in-law may have something worse. Syabusi finally asked the doctor tending his brother what is wrong. The doctor said the information is confidential and will not tell him. Neither will his brother. "My brother is not brave enough to tell me," says Syabusi, as he stares sadly toward the house next door, where his only sibling lies ill. "And I am not brave enough to ask him."

Kennedy Fugewane, a cheerful, elderly volunteer counselor, sits in an empty U.S.-funded clinic that offers fast, pinprick blood tests in Francistown, Botswana, pondering how to break through the

9

silence. This city suffers one of the world's highest infection rates, but people deny the disease because HIV is linked with sex. "We don't reveal anything," he says. "But people are so stigmatized even if they walk in the door." Africans feel they must keep private anything to do with sex. "If a man comes here, people will say he is running around," says Fugewane, though he acknowledges that men never do come. "If a woman comes, people will say she is loose. If anyone says they got HIV, they will be despised."

Pretoria University's Mary Crewe says, "It is presumed if you get AIDS, you have done something wrong." HIV labels you as living an immoral life. Embarrassment about sexuality looms more important than future health risks. "We have no language to talk candidly about sex," she says, "so we have no civil language to talk about AIDS." Volunteers like Fugewane try to reach out with flyers, workshops, youth meetings and free condoms, but they are frustrated by a culture that values its dignity over saving lives. "People here don't have the courage to come forward and say, 'Let me know my HIV status,'" he sighs, much less the courage to do something about it. "Maybe one day . . ."

Doctors bow to social pressure and legal strictures not to record AIDS on death certificates. "I write TB or meningitis or diarrhea but never AIDS," says South Africa's Dr. Moll. "It's a public document, and families would hate it if anyone knew." Several years ago, doctors were barred even from recording compromised immunity or HIV status on a medical file; now they can record the results of blood tests for AIDS on patient charts to protect other health workers. Doctors like Moll have long agitated to apply the same openness to death certificates. . . .

The Child in No. 17

In crib No. 17 of the spartan but crowded children's ward at the Church of Scotland Hospital in KwaZulu-Natal, a tiny, staring child lies dying. She is three and has hardly known a day of good health. Now her skin wrinkles around her body like an oversize suit, and her twig-size bones can barely hold her vertical as nurses search for a vein to take blood. In the frail arms hooked up to transfusion tubes, her veins have collapsed. The nurses palpate a threadlike vessel on the child's forehead. She mews like a wounded animal as one tightens a rubber band around her head to raise the vein. Tears pour unnoticed from her mother's eyes as she watches the needle tap-tap at her daughter's temple. Each time the whimpering child lifts a wan hand to brush away the pain, her mother gently lowers it. Drop by drop, the nurses manage to collect 1 cc of blood in five minutes.

The child in crib No. 17 has had TB, oral thrush, chronic diarrhea, malnutrition, severe vomiting. The vial of blood reveals her real ailment, AIDS, but the disease is not listed on her chart, and her mother says she has no idea why her child is so ill. She breast-fed her for two years, but once the little girl was weaned, she could not keep solid food down. For a long time, her mother thought something was wrong with the food. Now the child is afflicted with so many symptoms that her mother had to bring her to the hospital, from which sick babies rarely return.

She hopes, she prays her child will get better, and like all the mothers who stay with their children at the hospital, she tends her lovingly, constantly changing filthy diapers, smoothing sheets, pressing a little nourishment between listless lips, trying to tease a smile from the vacant, staring face. Her husband works in Johannesburg, where he lives in a men's squatter camp. He comes home twice a year. She is 25. She has heard of AIDS but does not know it is transmitted by sex, does not know if she or her husband has it. She is afraid this child will die soon, and she is afraid to have more babies. But she is afraid too to raise the subject with her husband. "He would not agree to that," she says shyly. "He would never agree to have no more babies."

Dr. Annick DeBaets, 32, is a volunteer from Belgium. In the two years she has spent here in Tugela Ferry, she has learned all about how hard it is to break the cycle of HIV transmission from mother to infant. The door to this 48-cot ward is literally a revolving one: sick babies come in, receive doses of rudimentary antibiotics, vitamins, food; go home for a week or a month; then come back as ill as ever. Most, she says, die in the first or second year. If she could just follow up with really intensive care, believes Dr. DeBaets, many of the wizened infants crowding three to a crib could live longer, healthier lives. "But it's very discouraging. We simply don't have the time, money or facilities for anything but minimal care."

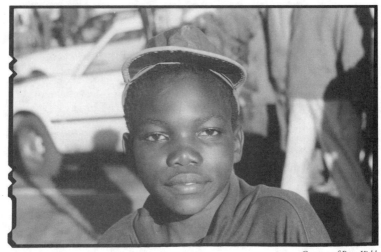

Courtesy of Pam Kidd

Much has been written about what South African Judge Edwin Cameron, himself HIV positive, calls his country's "grievous ineptitude" in the face of the burgeoning epidemic. Nowhere has that been more evident than in the government's failure to provide drugs that could prevent pregnant women from passing HIV to their babies. The government has said it can't afford the 300-rand-per-dose, 28-dose regimen of azt that neighboring nations like Botswana dole out, using funds and drugs from foreign donors. The late South African presidential spokesman Parks Mankahlana even suggested publicly that it was not cost effective to save these children when their mothers were already doomed to die: "We don't want a generation of orphans."

Yet these children—70,000 are born HIV positive in South Africa alone every year—could be protected from the disease for about $4 each with another simple, cheap drug called nevirapine. Until last month, the South African government steadfastly refused to license or finance the use of nevirapine despite the manufacturer's promise to donate the drug for five years, claiming that its "toxic" side effects are not yet known. This spring, however, the drug will finally be distributed to leading public hospitals in the country, though only on a limited basis at first.

The mother at crib No. 17 is not concerned with potential side effects. She sits on the floor cradling her daughter, crooning over and over, "Get well, my child, get well." The baby stares back without blinking. "It's sad, so sad, so sad," the mother says. The child died three days later.

The children who are left when parents die only add another complex dimension to Africa's epidemic. At 17, Tsepho Phale has been head of an indigent household of three young boys in the dusty township of Monarch, outside Francistown, for two years. He never met his father, his mother died of AIDS, and the grieving children possess only a raw concrete shell of a house. The doorways have no doors; the window frames no glass. There is not a stick of furniture. The boys sleep on piled-up blankets, their few clothes dangling from nails. In the room that passes for a kitchen, two paraffin burners sit on the dirt floor alongside the month's food: four cabbages, a bag of oranges and one of potatoes, three sacks of flour, some yeast, two jars of oil and two cartons of milk. Next to a dirty stack of plastic pans lies the mealy meal and rice that will provide their main sustenance for the month. A couple of bars of soap and two rolls of toilet paper also have to last the month. Tsepho has just brought these rations home from the social-service center where the "orphan grants" are doled out.

Tsepho has been robbed of a childhood that was grim even before his mother fell sick. She supported the family by "buying and selling things," he says, but she never earned more than a pittance. When his middle brother was knocked down by a car and left physically and mentally disabled, Tsepho's mother used the insurance money to build this house, so she would have one thing of value to leave her children. As the walls went up, she fell sick. Tsepho had to nurse her, bathe her, attend to her bodily functions, try to feed her. Her one fear as she lay dying was that her rural relatives would try to steal the house. She wrote a letter bequeathing it to her sons and bade Tsepho hide it.

As her body lay on the concrete floor awaiting burial, the relatives argued openly about how they would divide up the profits when they sold her dwelling. Tsepho gave the district commissioner's office the letter, preventing his mother's family from grabbing the house. Fine, said his relations; if you think you're a man, you look after your brothers. They have contributed nothing to the boys' welfare since. "It's as if we don't exist anymore either," says Tsepho. Now he struggles to keep house for the others, doing the cooking, cleaning, laundry and shopping.

The boys look at the future with despair. "It is very bleak," says Tsepho, kicking aimlessly at a bare wall. He had to quit school, has no job, will probably never get one. "I've given up my dreams. I have no hope."

Orphans have traditionally been cared for the African way: relatives absorb the children of the dead into their extended families. Some still try, but communities like Tsepho's are becoming saturated with orphans, and families can't afford to take on another kid, leaving thousands alone.

Now many must fend for themselves, struggling to survive. The trauma of losing parents is compounded by the burden of becoming a breadwinner. Most orphans sink into penury, drop out of school, suffer malnutrition, ostracism, psychic distress. Their makeshift households scramble to live on pitiful handouts—from overstretched relatives, a kind neighbor, a state grant—or they beg and steal in the streets. The orphans' present desperation forecloses a brighter future. "They hardly ever succeed in having a life," says Siphelile Kaseke, 22, a counselor at an AIDS orphans' camp near Bulawayo. Without education, girls fall into prostitution, and older boys migrate illegally to South Africa, leaving the younger ones to go on the streets.

Every day spent in this part of africa is acutely depressing: there is so little countervailing hope to all the stories of the dead and the doomed. "More than anywhere else in the world, AIDS in Africa was met with apathy," says Suzanne LeClerc-Madlala, a lecturer at the University of Natal. The consequences of the silence march on: infection soars, stigma hardens, denial hastens death, and the chasm between knowledge and behavior widens. The present disaster could be dwarfed by the woes that loom if Africa's epidemic rages on. The human losses could wreck the region's frail economies, break down civil societies and incite political instability.

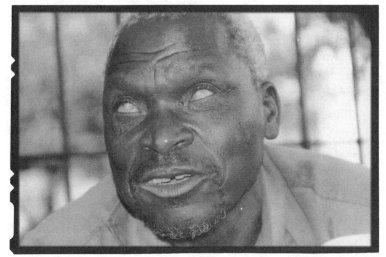

Courtesy of Pam Kidd

In the face of that, every day good people are doing good things. Like Dr. Moll, who uses his after-job time and his own fund raising to run an extensive volunteer home-care program in KwaZulu-Natal. And Busi Magwazi, who, along with dozens of others, tends the sick for nothing in the Durban-based Sinoziso project. And Patricia Bakwinya, who started her Shining Stars orphan-care program in Francistown with her own zeal and no money, to help youngsters like Tsepho Phale. And countless individuals who give their time and devotion to ease southern Africa's plight.

But these efforts can help only thousands; they cannot turn the tide. The region is caught in a double bind. Without treatment, those with HIV will sicken and die; without prevention, the spread of infection cannot be checked. Southern Africa has no other means available to break the vicious cycle, except to change everyone's sexual behavior—and that isn't happening.

The essential missing ingredient is leadership. Neither the countries of the region nor those of the wealthy world have been able or willing to provide it.

South Africa, comparatively well off, comparatively well educated, has blundered tragically for years. AIDS invaded just when apartheid ended, and a government absorbed in massive transition relegated the disease to a back page. An attempt at a national education campaign wasted millions on a farcical musical. The premature release of a local wonder drug ended in scandal when the drug turned out to be made of industrial solvent. Those fiascoes left the gov-

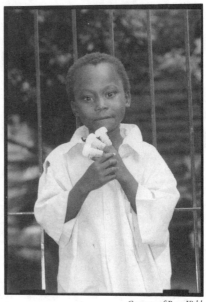

Courtesy of Pam Kidd

ernment skittish about embracing expensive programs, inspiring a 1998 decision not to provide azt to HIV-positive pregnant women. Zimbabwe too suffers savagely from feckless leadership. Even in Botswana, where the will to act is gathering strength, the resources to follow through have to come from foreign hands.

AIDS' grip here is so pervasive and so complex that all societies—theirs and ours—must rally round to break it. These countries are too poor to doctor themselves. The drugs that could begin to break the cycle will not be available here until global pharmaceutical companies find ways to provide them inexpensively. The health-care systems required to prescribe and monitor complicated triple-cocktail regimens won't exist unless rich countries help foot the bill. If there is ever to be a vaccine, the West will have to finance its discovery and provide it to the poor. The cure for this epidemic is not national but international.

The deep silence that makes African leaders and societies want to deny the problem, the corruption and incompetence that render them helpless is something the West cannot fix. But the fact that they are poor is not. The wealthy world must help with its zeal and its cash if southern Africa is ever to be freed of the AIDS plague.

NELSON MANDELA

Former President of South Africa

Care, Support and Destigmatization

Closing Statements at the XIV International AIDS Conference
Barcelona, Spain
July 12, 2002

Since last we came together at the Durban conference in 2000, we are told that six million more people have died as a result of HIV/AIDS. And, worst of all, that within the next twenty years seventy million people will die unless drastic action is taken. There are many issues that I would like to touch upon in these few words: issues of poverty and the burden of disease in developing countries, and the impact that this has on the AIDS pandemic; the importance of investment in developing countries to spur the economic growth which will ensure a sustained response to the epidemic; the importance of the community response to HIV/AIDS; and the rooting out of denial about the cause and consequences of AIDS.

In prevention of HIV infection in the youth, we have a remarkable initiative in South Africa called *loveLife*, which is a bold and ambitious attempt to reduce HIV infection by promoting: sexual health and a healthy future for young people; the extraordinary vulnerability of women to HIV infection and the importance of gender issues in the fight against AIDS; the importance of preventing the transmission of HIV infection from mother to child (AIDS should not be a disease of children!); the importance of finding the vaccine and of communities being prepared to participate in large-scale vaccine trials.

The list goes on and on, but we do not have time to address all of these important subjects. Instead, we have to select a few issues, which we currently regard as requiring the most urgent agenda. Nothing can be more heart-rending and in need of urgent attention than the case of AIDS orphans, who so often find themselves rejected and ostracized by communities.

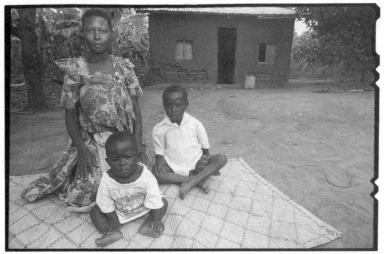

Courtesy of Jonathan W. Rodgers

Personally, nothing can shake me more than the sight of these innocent young children suffering physically, socially, and emotionally. There are nearly fourteen million children who have lost one or both parents to AIDS. It is predicted that there will be more than twenty-five million of them by 2010. This is a tragedy of enormous consequence. I'm sure you have been told that AIDS is killing more people than were killed by all the worst wars of history and natural disasters. AIDS is a war against humanity.

What we talk about, and the actions we take, must be influenced by the fact that this is a war, which requires mobilization of the entire population. These children will grow up without the love and care of their parents, and most of them will be deprived of their basic rights—shelter, food, health, and education. Many will be subjected to abuse, violence, exploitation, discrimination, trafficking, and loss of inheritance. We have an obligation to provide the proper care and support for these children. No adult can stand by and watch while these children suffer.

As adults, we have collective and individual responsibility to stop this now. The stigma and discrimination inflicted on these children are atrocious and inexcusable. Many people suffering from AIDS are not killed by the disease itself, but are killed by the stigma surrounding everybody who has HIV/AIDS.

That is why their leaders must do everything in their power to fight and to win the struggle against this stigma. Likewise, it is inexcusable to subject any person infected or affected by HIV/AIDS to such abuse and rejection. We must, therefore, tackle the stigma and discrimination associated with HIV/AIDS with even greater urgency. We must show that we care for all those affected by this terrible disease, and that we are doing something about it. Eloquence on this pandemic is good, but not sufficient. That is the first part of trying to direct the attention of the community to this pandemic, but what is more, what you do about it on the ground. Unless we are able to follow what you say by doing something practical to deal with this situation, our eloquence is less than useful.

When I was the President of South Africa, I went round the country together with the then-Minister of Social Welfare. Every city or rural area we went to, we told parents "bring the children who are suffering from terminal disease, like HIV/AIDS, cancer, tuberculosis, malaria. We also want you to bring children who are disabled, either physically or mentally." And the fact the president of the country is seen sitting at tables with children with HIV/AIDS and suffering from terminal diseases, children who are disabled, makes the parents less ashamed of their children. And it's certain.

Parents will say, *if the President of the country and the Minister of Welfare can sit at a table and enjoy a meal with our children, who suffer from terminal diseases, who are disabled, why must we be ashamed of them? We want them to come out and be seen, and to enjoy life like ordinary individuals.* Every year, I bring together between fifteen hundred and two thousand children, and I go right round the country. There is hardly any province in our country that has not seen this message I bring home. And that is how we give hope to children, who otherwise hardly have a future at all. It is very important for us, to go to the ground, and to tell the community how to deal with this pandemic.

I know, for example, a judge who sits in one of our highest courts, who has HIV/AIDS. He came to brief me about his position. His immune system was almost destroyed. He could not walk, but somehow he came to me, to fight back and win this battle. *This is the food that you must eat.* He followed that advice, and his immune system became stronger. He is now in the highest office in the highest court of the country. If a judge can do so, you also can do so.

But you must not be ashamed of speaking out and telling the community that *I suffer from HIV/AIDS.* In jail, I contracted TB. And, outside jail, I was found to be a cancer victim. My colleagues did not stigmatize me. They gave me all their love and support. There is no reason whatsoever why sufferers should hide that they have been affected by this pandemic. Because when you keep quiet—and this is something we have heard a hundred times—when you keep quiet, you are signing your own death warrant.

And the best thing to do is to practice. Say *I have this disease. I want to be cured.* We need to remind ourselves why so many of these children are orphans today: because their parents were not able to get access to treatment for AIDS, most likely because they could not afford it. Or because they lived in a country that was too poor to provide their basic health care. We must know that one of the greatest assaults to human dignity is poverty, where you wake up not knowing where you're going to get your next meal, where you cannot have decent accommodations for yourself and for your children, where you cannot feed them, where you cannot send them to the high school. That is the greatest assault on human dignity, and that is why we should pay particular attention to the poor who are ill, whose immune system is not capable of resisting these terminal diseases.

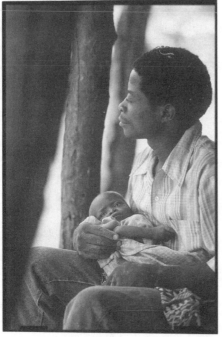
Courtesy of World Vision

I ask all leaders in the world: Is this acceptable? We know that there are treatments available that restore the immune system, stop the opportunistic infections, especially TB, and return an AIDS sufferer to good health, for several years, at least. Is it acceptable that these dying parents have no hope of access to treatment? The simple answer is no. We must find ways—we must find ways and means to make life-saving treatment available to all who need it. Regardless of whether they can pay for it, or where they live, or for any other reason, why should treatment be denied? If parents with AIDS can be given a few more years, perhaps several years or even longer, then their children will be given a much better opportunity for nurturing their survival and development.

Those few years of additional life will be the most precious for all of those parents and children. For those of us who are more fortunate than those dying parents, it is a timely reminder of the sanctity of human life. We should be prepared to give all that we have, give those families that are stricken by AIDS those extra few years. Nothing is better for your own well being than the feeling that *I am contributing practically towards those who are affected by this pandemic.*

In my country, I approach businesses and ask them to send children to school—high school, university. Generally, I arrange no less than three hundred scholarships per year. I arranged for a scholarship for a young lady of twenty to go to university. Her results on the tests for university were excellent. She attracted a lot of praise from her lecturers. Then, suddenly, she found that she had AIDS and went to the hospital. I was out of the country. And, because she could not pay the hospital charges, I came back and I immediately contacted her. And I asked her to come for lunch, knowing that she's an AIDS sufferer. I was then told, before I could enter the gate, to meet her at the gate. But after fifteen minutes, I asked, "Where are these people?"

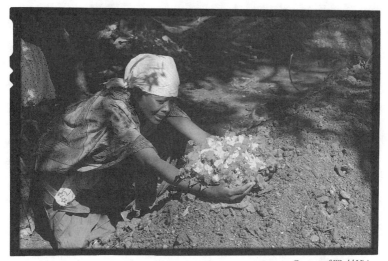

Courtesy of World Vision

Eventually, she came with her parents. She could hardly walk, and I said, "just go straight to the table." . . . And very sadly, had to go from here straight to hospital. And my secretary immediately phoned the hospital, and the doctor in charge told me that there is very little that we can do.

I was devastated. And within a week, because they couldn't do anything, they discharged her. My wife and I went to see her. Then we arranged for her to have drugs, to have good food. Then I phoned about two weeks later, and a very sharp, strong voice replied. I said, "Who is speaking?" She gave me the name—same girl. I said, "I can't believe that!" She was now strong, and my secretary, without even consulting me, had got her new pajamas and a new dressing gown.

I have raised more than 800,000 rand for her, and I send her some money every month so that she can eat properly, she can get all the drugs that she needs. I first sent her 500 rand a month, but my wife almost left me in disgust. And she said, "We must give her R2,000 a month." That's what she said.

One of the members of my staff took this money to her, and she had taken the R500 before. She said, I came across a new person, I can't believe that it's the same girl who was written off by the doctors. She is now recovered. There is life after HIV/AIDS.

I have three challenges to put to the world today. The first is to challenge all institutions, public and private, and all their leaders, to make a start on treatment access today, and to make rapid and real progress in achieving access to AIDS treatment for all those who need it—wherever they may be in the world, regardless of whether they can afford to pay or not. We place such a huge emphasis on treatment, quite simply, because treatment will provide hope for the future.

The great tragedy of HIV infection is that most people, surely more than 90 percent, do not know that they are infected with the virus. They continue, unwittingly, to spread the infection. With the hope of treatment, people will have a reason to go for HIV counseling and testing, but, it must be on an entirely voluntary and confidential basis.

Businesses must stop humiliating people and testing them openly whether they have HIV or not. All that is required is to talk to people, constantly, to say, "If you don't go for testing, if you have got AIDS and you don't know about it, you are signing your own death warrant. The only way in which you can be saved is if you go for a test, and then accept what the doctor says to you." I believe that this is the single most important prevention tool that we have, because it is the one that is most likely to change behavior.

My second challenge today is to all individuals: you need to establish where you stand in the fight against HIV/AIDS, and you can only do this by being aware of your HIV status. For those of you who are HIV positive, there is hope. You can live with HIV, and the rest of the world cares about you.

The sooner you establish your HIV status, the more you can do for yourself, and the more that can be done for you by others. And if voluntary counseling and testing is not available free of charge where you live, then you must demand it. It is your right to know.

My final challenge today is to the leaders of this world. There is no doubt that strong leadership is the key to an effective response in the war against AIDS. Leadership starts at the top. When the top person is committed, the response is much more effective—this means not only political leaders, but also business leaders, union leaders, religious leaders, traditional leaders, and the leaders of NGOs.

One has to make special mention of the role played by NGOs and the leadership in those organizations. These are often small organizations with meager resources that have made an impact far beyond what would have been expected from their size. One is often moved to reflect that, if only the big institutions of government and business had made a similar effort proportionately, we might very well already have turned the tide of the AIDS pandemic.

In this regard, the Bill and Melinda Gates Foundation and other big companies have done very well, by making funds available for us to treat this pandemic. Now, many people are criticizing big business and governments because they are not doing sufficiently. That is one part of it, it is true. But the other part, which many people don't talk about, is our own shortcomings. We have not developed proper strategies to get the money out of them.

President Clinton will tell you that as facilitator in Burundi, I asked him for money. He gave it to me on the spot. That money got finished. I went back to the President of the United States, George Bush, and I said, *I want a million dollars*. He gave it to me.

I have gone back to almost every continent and asked for money. For my organization, in Africa alone, I collected sixty-six million dollars, and you know how poor Africa is. In the Middle East, I collected seventy-three million dollars, and in Asia, eighty-nine million for my organization, the ANC.

Now, I was discussing this morning about the complaints against government, and I was saying, let us look at the strategy that we're using, because if we corrected ourselves, we would be able to succeed more than we do. One of the most difficult things in life is not just to influence others; it is to change your own character.

And we are required to do that today in fighting this pandemic. We must correct our own mistakes. It is good to criticize governments when they are stingy, but you need to do much more than criticize. I have criticized government openly, but I've gone to the same government I've criticized, and I've said, *Can you put money in my hand?*

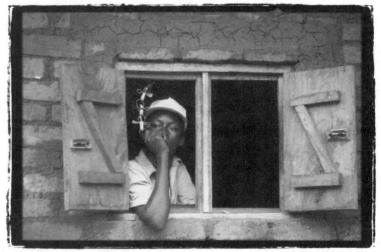

Courtesy of Jonathan W. Rodgers

People, brave and courageous men and women, let us not be afraid to criticize and speak up, but, at the same time, let's not be afraid to go to the same people that we criticize and say, *We have this particular problem; can you give us money?*

But our own strategy must be changed. We have great appreciation for the courageous leadership given by many in all sectors of society, in different parts of the world. At the same time, I wish to repeat the appeal and challenge I have so often made, calling on all leaders in the world today to ask themselves what they have personally done to help diminish the impact of the AIDS pandemic. And whatever they have done, or have not done, to commit themselves to doing more from today. As one who has led almost the entirety of his life in a struggle to build a better world, often against odds that were thought insurmountable, I want to say to all of you who are activists in the war against AIDS, you have my greatest admiration. Keep on fighting, and you will overcome the terrible scourge of human kind.

In Africa, we have a concept known as *ubuntu*, based on the recognition that we are only people because of other people. We are all human, and the HIV/AIDS epidemic affects us all in the end. If we discard the people who are dying from AIDS, then we can no longer call ourselves people.

The time to act is now. We can make a difference. I thank you.

Reprinted by permission of The Nelson Mandela Foundation.

WILLIAM H. FRIST, M.D.

United States Senator

Taking Our Stand Against HIV/AIDS
July 24, 2002

A Plague of Biblical Proportions

I spent the first twenty years of my career studying and working in medicine. I graduated from medical school in 1978. After that, I trained as a surgical resident for eight years. I then worked as a heart and lung transplant surgeon until I was elected to the United States Senate in 1994. During that time, HIV/AIDS went from a disease without a name to a global pandemic claiming nearly twenty million people infected.

It's hard to imagine an organism that cannot survive outside the human body yet can take such an immense toll on human life. But HIV/AIDS has done just that—already killing thirteen million people. Today more than forty million people—including three million children—are infected with HIV/AIDS. HIV/AIDS is a plague of biblical proportions.

And it has only begun to wreak its destruction upon humanity. Though one person dies from AIDS every ten seconds, two people are infected with HIV in that same period of time. If we continue to fight HIV/AIDS in the future as we have in the past, it will kill sixty-eight million people in the forty-five most affected countries between the years 2000 and 2020. We are losing the battle against this disease.

There is neither a cure nor a vaccine for HIV/AIDS. But we do have reliable and inexpensive means to test for it. Also, because we know how the disease is spread, we know how to prevent it from being spread. We even have treatments that can suppress the virus to almost undetectable levels and significantly reduce the risk of mothers infected with HIV/AIDS from passing the disease to their children.

We have many tools at our disposal to fight the spread of HIV/AIDS. But are we using those tools as effectively as possible? The gloomy statistics prove overwhelmingly that we are not. What we must do is focus on what is truly needed and what is proven to work, and marshal resources towards those solutions. We have beaten deadly diseases on a global scale before; we can win the battle against HIV/AIDS too.

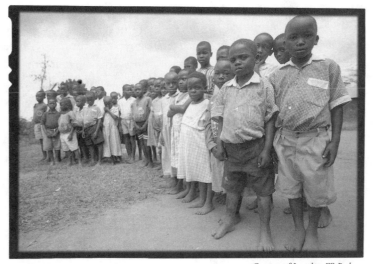

Courtesy of Jonathan W. Rodgers

A Global Problem Requires Global Leadership

More than 70 percent of people infected with HIV/AIDS worldwide live in Sub-Saharan Africa. But the devastation of the disease—and its potential to devastate in the future—is by no means limited to Africa. HIV/AIDS is global and lapping against the shores of even the most advanced and developed nations in the world.

Asia and the Pacific are home to 6.6 million people infected with HIV/AIDS—including one million of the five million people infected last year. Infections are rising sharply—especially among the young and injecting drug users—in Russia and other Eastern European countries. And the Americas are not immune. Six percent of adults in Haiti and 4 percent of adults in the Bahamas are infected with HIV/AIDS.

I believe the United States must lead the global community in the battle against HIV/AIDS. As Sir Elton John said in testimony before a committee on which I serve in the United States Senate, "What America has done for its people has made America strong. What America has done for others has made America great." Perhaps in no better way can the United States show its greatness in the 21st century—and show its true selflessness to other nations—than leading a victorious effort to halt the spread of HIV/AIDS.

But solving a global problem requires global leadership. International organizations, national governments, faith-based organizations, and the private sector must coordinate with each other and work together toward common goals. And, most importantly, we must make communities the focus of our efforts. Though global leadership must come from places like Washington, New York, and Brussels, resources must be directed to where they are needed the most—to the men and women in the villages and clinics and schools fighting HIV/AIDS on the front lines.

Significant and Sustainable Progress

Adequate funding is and will remain crucial to winning the battle against HIV/AIDS. But just as crucial as the amount of funding is how it is spent. Should we spend on programs that prevent or lower the rate of infection? Should we spend on treatments that may prolong the life of those who are already infected? Should we spend on the research and development of a vaccine? The answer is *yes* . . . to all three questions.

We can only win the battle against HIV/AIDS with a balanced approach of prevention, care, and treatment, and the research and development of an effective vaccine. HIV/AIDS has already infected tens of millions of people and will infect tens of millions more. We need to support proven strategies that will slow the spread of the virus and offer those already infected with the opportunity to live as normal lives as possible. And if our goal is to eradicate HIV/AIDS—and I believe that is an eminently achievable goal—then we must develop a highly effective vaccine.

But even with proven education programs, or free access to anti-retroviral drugs, or a vaccine that is 80 to 90 percent effective, our ability to slow the spread of HIV/AIDS and treat those already infected would be hampered. The infrastructure to battle HIV/AIDS in the most affected areas is limited at best. We need to train health-care workers, help build adequate health facilities, and distribute basic lab and computer equipment to make significant and sustainable progress over the long-term.

Not Only the Disease Itself

To win the battle against HIV/AIDS, we must not only fight the disease itself, but also underlying conditions that contribute to its spread—poverty, starvation, civil unrest, limited access to health-care, meager education systems and reemerging infectious diseases. Stronger societies, stronger economies, and stronger democracies will facilitate a stronger response to HIV/AIDS and ensure a higher quality of life in the nations most affected by and most vulnerable to the disease and its continued spread.

And we can make significant progress without vast sums of money and burgeoning new programs. Take, for example, providing something as basic and essential as access to clean water. Three hundred million, or 45 percent of, people in Sub-Saharan Africa don't have access to clean water. And those who are fortunate enough to have access sometimes spend hours walking to and from a well or spring.

It costs only one thousand dollars to build a "spring box" that provides access to natural springs and protects against animal waste run-off and other elements that may cause or spread disease. Eighty-five percent of the ten million people who live in Uganda don't have access to a nearby supply of clean water. It would cost only twenty-five million dollars to build enough spring boxes to provide most of the people living in rural Uganda with nearby access to clean water.

Providing access to clean water is just one of the many ways in which the global community can empower the people most affected by and most vulnerable to HIV/AIDS. In some cases, such efforts—like supporting democracy and encouraging free mar-kets—may cost little but will make a significant difference in the battle against HIV/AIDS and the quality of life of billions of people throughout the world.

Our Stand Against HIV/AIDS

We have defeated infectious diseases before—sometimes on even larger scale. Smallpox, for example, killed 300 million people in the 20th century. And as late as the 1950s, it afflicted up to fifty million people per year. But by 1979, smallpox was officially eradicated thanks to an aggressive and concerted global effort.

What if we had not launched that effort in 1967? What if we had waited another thirty-five years? Smallpox likely would have infected 350 million and killed forty million more people. That is a hefty price for inaction—a price that we should be grateful we did not pay then, and we should not want to pay now.

Right now we are losing the battle against HIV/AIDS. But that doesn't mean we can't win it in the end. Indeed, I believe we will ultimately eradicate HIV/AIDS. We have the tools to slow the spread of the disease and provide treatment to those already infected. And we have the scientific knowledge to develop an effective vaccine. But we need to focus our resources on what is truly needed and what is proven to work. And we need global leadership to meet a global challenge.

In 2020, when it is estimated that more than 85 million people will have died from HIV/AIDS, how will we look back upon this

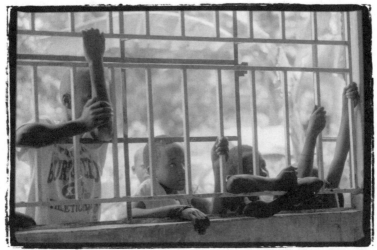

Courtesy of Jonathan W. Rodgers

day? Will we have proven the experts right with inaction? Or will we have proven them wrong with initiative? I hope that we will be able to say that in the year 2002 we took our stand against HIV/AIDS and began to turn back what could have been, but never became the most deadly disease in the history of the world.

Written for The aWAKE Project,
Copyright © 2002 by Sen. William H. Frist, M.D.

MARY GRAHAM

President of Women of Faith

Help Me Be Like You

AIDS is a global problem, and it affects us all whether we know it or not. What once seemed an isolated issue has become a challenge for the whole world. Especially the church.

There was a time when everything I knew about AIDS was in a textbook or a movie. Sometimes a headline in the newspaper was bold and caught my attention, but I don't think I ever made it through the whole article. Ashamedly, I admit it didn't seem essential information for me. It applied to people in a sub-culture in my own world, or in another world far from my own. Through the years, my indifference has changed dramatically to both care and genuine grief.

Last year while traveling abroad with World Vision on behalf of Women of Faith, I visited an HIV/AIDS clinic. I was not prepared for what I saw. The rooms were filled with women, mostly very young. Some had small children who were also HIV positive. Others were in full blown, final stages of the dreaded disease. Some looked healthy but were walking around with a death sentence flowing through their veins.

As I met and talked with each of these women, I felt more and more compassion for their need and passion to scream at the top of my voice, *Somebody do something!* In a nutshell, the stories went something like this: Young girls, from the ages of eight or ten, had been sold into prostitution by families needing money for life's basic essentials. The women were sold again and again by their "masters," becoming sexual pawns, held hostage to the dirt-cheap desires of men. Ultimately, they became infected with the disease, and gave birth to fatherless children who were born with the infection. Then, as young adults, they were tossed aside as rubbish.

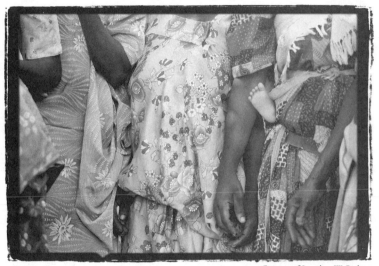

Courtesy of Jonathan W. Rodgers

I thought about all the discussions and stimulating conversations I'd had through the years with friends regarding "a woman's choice," and I felt heartsick. Regardless of who we are or what we believe in America, our 'choices' are myriad. I couldn't get my heart and mind past these desperate women and their need. They had never had a choice of any kind, and they have none now. My heart was broken, which was God's gift to me.

A recent headline in *USA Today* took my breath away, "AIDS to Orphan 25 Million." Think of it. We cannot bear to think of one child losing her mother. Twenty five million motherless children? And of those, many carry the virus themselves. This is not an isolated issue—nothing remote about it, and it will not solve itself. As has been the case for twenty years, it will get worse and worse. Who will help? Who will do something?

It has to be the church. We must be on the leading edge of those who care. Jesus clearly called us to this kind of action. He burdens our hearts for the needs of others, gives us grace to care, hope that makes a difference, and the courage to step up to the plate, even when the need is overwhelming.

He is the one who ignored the prejudice of his culture and reached out to those who were rejected and forsaken. Religious leaders—right and left—in the time of Christ were making pronouncements about the lack of responsibility of the church and its people. "Wrong!" Jesus seemed to say. Out of his compassionate heart, he looked beyond what was easily perceived, to the deeper issues of the plight of people. He touched the outcasts, the lepers, and those unable to help themselves. He went about doing good. He helped and it changed lives.

And he's the one we follow. Unfortunately, many of us have not just been oblivious to the problem of AIDS worldwide, including our own country, we've been objectionable to it. We've felt offended, critical, judgmental, and averse to the issue. The problem is, it's not just an "issue." It is people we're talking about. People are hurting and dying now by the millions.

I personally know many believers who have given their lives to this cause. They work every day somewhere in the world nurturing and caring for those whose lives are ravished by this plague. Their work is saving lives, protecting women and children, and they are being the tangible love of Christ to those who suffer. Millions have secured life eternally because someone cared enough to do what Christ would do. May God give them grace in abundance.

Last year in that clinic there was a woman whose face glowed like the Shekinah Glory—it was as if the divine presence of Christ was in her countenance. Although only in her early twenties, Lydia will live just a few more years. As her story unfolded, we realized her entire life had been spent being tossed from one garbage heap to another . . . until now. With the love of Christ, someone brought her to this safe place. She found love, kindness, and peace. In addition, there was provision for her physical needs. She sang with a little choir at the clinic and even when she was singing she never stopped smiling. She said to me, "I am so lucky." I cried.

I remembered the words of Isaiah, "Whom shall I send and who will go for me?" I silently prayed that the Lord would help me know what to do. Anyone in my place that day would have responded as I did. The love of Christ 'constrained' me, and it would you. I challenge you to get in touch with the reality of the AIDS crises. It is a global problem and cannot be dismissed. Ask God to give you his concern for those whose lives are broken by the disease. Pray boldly that he will give you some personal contribution to make. Frankly, one of the most important first steps is that our hearts will be tender about this emergency. That could be the most crucial turning point for the church. And then do something. Do *something*. As Christians we know there are three things to consider: we can pray, or give, or go. Or all three. Nobody can do everything. But everybody can do something. If we won't, who will?

Oh, God, give me your heart for these who suffer. Protect me from ignorance, indifference and hostile, judgmental statements. Help me be a part of the solution. Help me be like you.

Written for The aWAKE Project,
Copyright © 2002 by Mary Graham.

DESMOND TUTU

Archbishop of South Africa

Christmas Sermon

Washington National Cathedral
December 25, 1999

I wish you all who are gathered in this beautiful Cathedral Church of St. Peter and Paul, and you who are sharing in this act of worship through television, a joyous and blessed Christmas—the last of this century. In doing this, we commemorate herewith an event that took place nearly 2000 years ago, actually nineteen hundred and

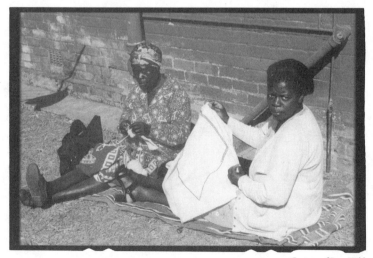

Courtesy of Pam Kidd

ninety-nine years ago. It was a momentous event, truly indeed epoch making. We commemorate the birth of a baby whose coming into the world helped mark the ages—everything before this birth belonged in the B.C. era, the time before this Christ child, and everything afterwards was identified as A.D., Anno Domino, the year of the Lord, to whom all times belonged. Can you imagine what Hollywood would have done, given a free hand with such a momentous event? We can imagine the spectacular extravaganza in Technicolor that would have resulted!

That beautiful Christmas carol "O Little Town of Bethlehem" says so poignantly, "How silently, how silently, the wondrous gift was given." God, the ever-courteous Lord, would not wish to violate our integrity by the kind of evidence that would nullify our precious freedom to choose. And so God, the omnipotent One, possessing all, because God created it all, came, not in a blinding glory that would make faith superfluous but as a vulnerable little infant, nuzzled by the animals. For this Divine Royal Child was born not in a royal palace, not even in the local inn, but in a stable, for there was no room for him in the inn. If someone had asked, "Who is that baby?" could anyone really have said, "Oh, that is God!"

Cape Town in South Africa is famous for its beauty and is also famous for its graffiti. When I was Archbishop, near the Archbishop's official residence, *Bishopscourt,* these words appeared on a wall: "I was an Episcopalian until I put two and two together." In a way, we could say Jesus is God's graffiti, to say to each one of us, every single one, "I love you with a love that cannot change." And God speaks those words, quietly, gently into your heart, into my heart, into the hearts of all of us. Stevie Wonder used to have a hit that said, "I just called to say I love you." In Jesus, in this birth, it is as if God were saying to you, and to you, and to you, and to me, "I just called to say I love you. You are special to me; you are precious."

Through this Christmas event, God was saying too, "I am a biased God, a God who takes sides. I am biased in favor of the weak, of the vulnerable, of the voiceless. I am biased in favor of the sinner so that in my heaven, there is not just joy, but greater joy over one sinner who repents, than over ninety-nine needing no repentance. I have a soft spot for the despised, the ostracized."

Just look at the parents God chose for his Son. They did not have clout even to get a room in the inn. Somebody says Joseph went to the innkeeper and said, "Please, please help me, my wife is pregnant," and the innkeeper replied, "It's not my fault." And Joseph retorted, "It's not mine either." It was such as these who were to become his friends, the prostitutes, the tax collectors, the scum of society. It was about these that he could say, so remarkably, "Inasmuch as you have done it to the least of these, my sisters and my brothers, you have done it to me."

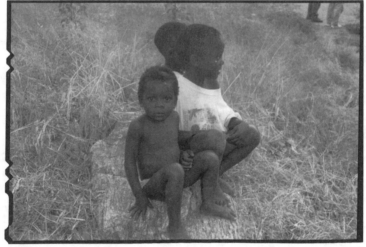

Courtesy of Pam Kidd

In his coming, in his turning an epoch to make it belong to the Lord, A.D., he proclaimed that all were God's children, all were members of one family—this new society ruled by kingdom values—love, compassion, gentleness, caring, and sharing and ruled by the ethic of family. That was truly revolutionary, truly radical. Wouldn't it still be in our world today, if we recognized that we were sisters and brothers, members of one family? Would we spend obscene amounts on defense budgets of death and destruction when a small amount would insure a good life for our sisters and brothers everywhere? They would have clean water, good education, and affordable health care. Would we wonder what to do with budget surpluses when our sisters and brothers were starving elsewhere—were dying of curable, preventable disease elsewhere?

If we knew ourselves to be sisters and brothers, would we allow members of our family in developing countries to carry huge burdens of un-payable debt? Would we not all support the Jubilee 2000 campaign to cancel international debt to give them a chance to make a new beginning in the new millennium? God through Jesus says to you, "I love you. You are precious to me and help me to have a truly Anno Domino in 2000—a new society, compassionate and gentle, caring, and sharing—for I just called to say I love you."

Amen.

Reprinted by permission of Lynn C. Franklin Associates, Ltd.
on behalf of the author.

MARGARET BECKER

Recording Artist

Hope for the Hopeless

I guess what stood out to me when I first arrived in the Mathari Valley was the absolute hopelessness. Everywhere, the brown dirt was littered with cardboard and tin.

The windows of our UN SUV were closed, their panes so hot we couldn't touch them. It was at least one hundred degrees outside. Reality seemed skewed as we passed the desperate sights. It was as if we were watching a television show, where the windows were television screens. It was all in front of us, but in some odd way we were not entirely responsible to it, because we were passing through. We would go to a hotel that night in the city. We would go home at the end of the week. *We* only had to look only for a little while.

We didn't even have to get out of the car if we didn't want to.

We drove for what seemed like a half-hour at least, through the tiny dirt roads lined with people and lean-tos. People sitting in the dirt, watching us pass in our white vehicle; watching with no expression. Neither interest nor disdain. Nothingness.

I was in Kenya with an organization that has been in the business of offering relief to the world for fifty years, through education and intervention: World Vision.

We were to have a police escort this morning, but fires broke out in this squatter settlement and all the officials were battling it. Police are necessary to prevent kidnappings of foreigners. We were told to stay close together and be aware of our surroundings.

Mile upon mile of families, some twelve and thirteen people, huddled on small clusters of dirt that they considered "theirs." True squatters, someone was designated to remain at all times, otherwise others would come and assume ownership. Some of the luckier among the people had corrugated steel panels that were leaned against one another to create a makeshift tent or wall. The toilet for all was a small gully the size of a gutter that was etched into the middle of the dirt road.

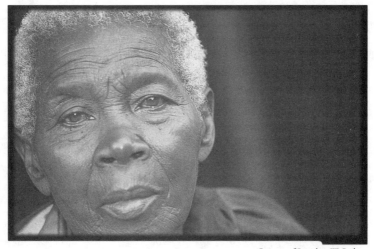

Courtesy of Jonathan W. Rodgers

I watched it pass from the relative comfort of the truck. I knew what I was seeing, but it didn't penetrate, even though I'd braced myself for the reality of it all before I ever arrived in Africa. World Vision warned me of what I might see: extreme poverty, desperate sickness, deformities caused by simple things like zinc deficiencies, so many hopeless situations. They told me, but I still wasn't prepared. How could I be? There is no reference here in my world. We have poverty, but for the most part not like this.

All week long we saw how the tiniest of interventions, like educating adults on the necessity of clean water, had changed the settlement for the better, saving lives from inane deaths caused by diarrhea.

At one project, a simple education on how to sew saved sixty women a year from prostitution—one of the more commonplace occupations for women in the Third World. But with organizations like World Vision, these Kenyan ladies were offered alternatives. I hovered in their little workshop, happy for the hope I felt. These women had a plan. They had simple resources, and their whole lives would be different now—in a better way. A future for these families, a future that we would despise according to our standards, but that was more than they could have ever hoped for.

Two days into the visit we went to the trash piles, the place where Nairobi dumps all of its urban garbage. The stench was overwhelming, burning the eyes. Hills upon hills of garbage heaps, with, of all things, people perched atop them. Babies, without shoes or clothing, barely able to walk, sifting through the piles for anything with which they can barter. A piece of wire that can be twisted to make a bracelet. A half eaten meal—anything. Our Kenyan guide explained the lack of adults on the pile.

"The hospital puts its trash here too. They do not dispose of their used utensils in any special way; they just toss them here. Of course you know about our problem with AIDS. These people here on the trash actually live there. Some never come down for their entire lives because if they leave, someone will take their place.

"The adults and the babies are mostly AIDS infected, from pricking themselves on the needles leftover from the hospital, and then —as adults will do—having sexual intercourse."

We stared. A baby forced his tiny hand into a smoldering opening in the heap about thirty feet up.

The guide spanned the vista; jaw set deep in thought. He turned to us finally and simply said, "AIDS is our biggest problem."

The last place we stopped on our tour was the AIDS Orphan Day Program. We walked into the tiny mud building to a group of children all wearing white t-shirts with the words *AIDS Orphan* printed on the front in English.

The fact that they wore anything declaring that they were connected to AIDS was shocking. In America, we've been so long averse to even discussing it, hiding behind the false veil of a "lifestyle" connection. To say *AIDS* was akin to saying *homosexual*. People felt free of any responsibility because it wasn't *their* problem. They led *good* lives.

Yet here, from infants to adolescents, were *children*, wearing these shirts that plainly spoke of their situation.

There was no shame. They had a disease. It was a tragic disease that would eventually kill them. That was it.

Our guide explained how the parents and their aunts and uncles had died of AIDS. It is almost wiping out an entire generation, leaving only the very young and the very old.

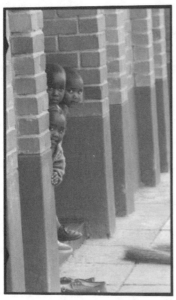

Courtesy of Pam Kidd

Grandparents who had long since raised their children—most times with great difficulty, now were forced to re-enter the fight to survive, to provide for their children's children. Some of them began with six children of their own. Now they were caring for multitudes, in some cases, more than twenty—with no house, no food, no source of income.

There are more than thirteen million of these children now. *Thirteen million.*

A small boy came up to me as I considered these things. He reached his arms out to me, and I picked him up.

There we were, two living breathing people, looking into one another's eyes. His shy smile convicted me and challenged me to forget everything I thought I knew about our world and how it works, about what is fair and not fair, about social stigmas and prejudices. It challenged me to find a way—*make* a way—to help the people I come in contact with *see him*. Just one person who will die a terrible death very soon, just one small boy who smiles, because he has a tee-shirt, and some food, and people who will hold him up from time to time.

I couldn't retreat behind the glass any longer. Standing in a continent where some rates of infection are as high as 35 percent—one third of the population in some countries.

I thought of the national study done by World Vision that showed how Christians feel about this issue, and mourned. I vowed that I would not be one of the 61 percent of who will not help overseas AIDS prevention and education programs. I *wouldn't* be one of the 54 percent who openly admit that they will do nothing to help. I did not have the luxury of turning a blind eye, because I held a boy in my arms. Just a boy. *Only* a boy.

A boy whose parents didn't know that unprotected sex was deadly. A boy whose mother or father received tainted blood, or stepped on a needle—just *people* living out *human lives*, with all the dramatic and mundane situations that we *all* face.

World Vision has helped me to help. They've been intervening in the African AIDS crisis since 1990. They couldn't ignore it then, when the rest of Christian America could. And now, as the epidemic threatens to affect our lives in every area from our economy to our health, I hope that we will all rise to the challenge—the way Jesus himself would.

I hope we get out of the car, walk in the unlovely places and begin picking people up one by one, changing the world, one person at a time.

And I pray that we do it all in the name of the greatest hope, our merciful, loving God, Jesus Christ.

Written for The aWAKE Project,
Copyright © 2002 by Margaret Becker.

JIMMY CARTER

Former President of the United States of America

Faith-based Groups Confronting HIV/AIDS
March 2002

It was almost twenty-four years ago when I first came to this great country, and when I arrived in Lagos I was met by my friend, President Obasanjo. The first thing he said was, "I have one request to make of you," and I immediately thought of the advanced weapons systems that my country had to sell, and if that wasn't the request I figured that he was going to ask for more USAID funds to come to Nigeria. But his request was, "I want you to join me tomorrow morning, Sunday, in helping with a religious service."

He hasn't changed, but the world has changed. One thing that we do at the Carter Center is to analyze all the conflicts in the world. There are now about 110 on our list, about seventy of which erupt into violence every year. Thirty of them are major wars. We analyze the causes of these conflicts and what might be done to prevent or to end them. It is very disturbing to me as a Christian to know that many of these wars are caused by religious belief.

Last Sunday my wife and I were in Sudan, a great nation torn apart for the last nineteen years by a terrible conflict that has cost more than two million lives. And the war is caused primarily by religious differences.

I have thought this morning about things that do not divide us but that bind us together. There are many faiths in this world with which we're familiar, but I think there is one common commitment, whether you are Hindu, or Buddhist, or Muslim, or Christian—Protestant or Catholic—and that is we pledge ourselves to have mercy and compassion and to alleviate the suffering of the poor.

You see the assignment given to me this morning if you read your bulletin. I've been in a quandary about how to address this issue in a church. If I were home in Plains, Georgia, I would be teaching the Bible. I do this every Sunday. And I've tried to think about the Christian approach in a church on Sunday morning to HIV/AIDS, and my only recourse really has been to turn to the example set for us by our Savior, Jesus Christ. How did Jesus address the question of sex and the violation of the Ten Commandments, "Thou shalt not commit adultery"? I've thought about the Samaritan woman at the well, who Christ pointed out had five lovers, none of them her husband. And I've thought about Mary Magdalene, the first woman to go into the empty tomb on Easter Sunday, and who became really the first missionary because she went and told the disciples about the risen Christ—and she was guilty of seven serious sins certainly including that of adultery. We know how Jesus reacted to those women.

But I think that the most vivid demonstration of that is found in John 8, beginning with the seventh verse, where a woman was brought to Christ by the arrogant political and religious leaders of the day. She had been caught in the act of adultery, and the penalty assigned to her by the law was execution by stoning. And to trap Christ, they said, "How do you treat this woman?" Jesus looked at her, and he looked at her accusers, and he leaned down, the Bible says, and wrote some words in the sand. And he looked up and said that, "He who is without sin cast the first stone." And one by one her accusers walked away, and then Christ looked at her and said, "Go and sin no more."

This is, I think, pertinent to the AIDS question. I think another story comes to us from Luke 12, where ten lepers came to Jesus and asked him to cure their affliction. I would equate lepers in those days with AIDS victims today. Luke 17:12 is where it begins.

A leper was an outcast, feared by all the citizens who saw him. They had to identify themselves by their dress and also by crying out, "I am a leper, I am a leper," when everyone came near them. They were not only looked upon as sick and contagious, but the general presumption, never disputed, was that they had leprosy because they were sinful, that this was a punishment imposed upon them by God. How did Christ react to this abomination for these outcasts and despised people? He healed them. And told them to go and be cleansed in the law so that they could live a normal life. It is interesting that only one came back to thank Christ. He happened to be a despised Samaritan.

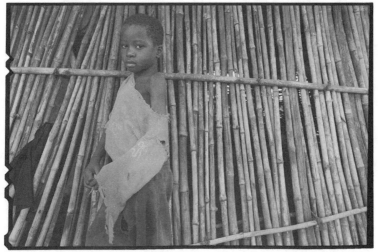

Courtesy of World Vision

How do we fortunate people, we rich people, we blessed and secure people, react to this blight of AIDS on the world? We have 900,000 AIDS sufferers in my country. We spend ten billion dollars each year on this problem, which if you figure it out is about ten thousand U.S. dollars per patient. You have 3.6 million HIV-positive people in Nigeria. Health is under reasonable control by the enlightened and dynamic and aggressive leadership of your president. We came earlier this week from another country, which I won't

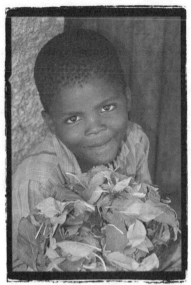
Courtesy of World Vision

name, where the president has avoided this responsibility completely, and AIDS is rampant and growing every day. Nigeria is blessed by this leadership, but we have to remember that our duties don't just go to admiring a president or hoping the governors and ministers will take a stance against this terrible affliction.

Some day we Christians, perhaps all people, will be judged by the sovereign and gentle Christ. If you look in the 25th chapter of Matthew you will find that Jesus says, *I will be the judge and you will be standing before me and divided into two groups, one is a sheep and one is a goat. The sheep will be those who ministered to me when I was on earth. When I was sick you came and helped me; when I was hungry, you fed me; when I was thirsty, you gave me drink; when I was in prison, you visited me.* And the people said Lord, *When did I ever have a chance to give you food or water or visit you?* And he said, *As you have done it unto the least of these my brothers you have done it unto me.* And he looked at the goats who were very proud people. They thought they were naturally in a superior position. They had attended church every Sunday and sung hymns and enjoyed the services and ostentatiously been Christians. And he said, *When I was sick you didn't visit me, you didn't give me food and water.* And they said, *Lord, we would have done anything for you.* He said, *As you did not do it unto the least of these, you did not do it unto me.*

Christ was merciful. There would be no way that I would stand in a Christian church and say it's satisfactory or godlike or permissible to have any sex except for the one person whom we have chosen for our life's partner. The Bible says, "Thou shalt not commit adultery," and Jesus said not one jot or tittle of that law will be changed. But we know that people sin, *All have sinned and come short of the glory of God,* the Bible says. We know that our God is one of forgiveness and grace and mercy and love.

So we should minister to those who commit sexual sins, casual sex, extramarital sex, even adultery, betraying wives or husbands. There is a simple way for those who violate marital laws to prevent having AIDS. We all know what it is; it's been publicized. The Gates and we were with commercial sex workers yesterday morning, lovely young women, who sell their bodies ten to fifteen times a day, they told us, for money. They know how to prevent having AIDS, and everyone in this country knows.

But we should remember that there is an example set for us by Jesus Christ, for those who go astray, for those who are despised, for those who suffer because of their own sins, for those who are outcasts, for those who are poor. We call ourselves Christians, sometimes casually. We fail to remember what the word *Christian* means. It means little Christ. And when we think about being or claiming to be a little Christ, the responsibility in alleviating the suffering or preventing the suffering of others becomes much more vivid and personal in our minds.

So my message this morning, in summary, about HIV/AIDS is for us try to be little Christs. And to deal aggressively and benevolently with love and compassion, sharing our wealth to make sure that the ignorant, the poor, the outcast, are prevented from having this terrible disease. My belief is that that is the world of My Savior, Jesus Christ.

Jimmy Carter and Bill Gates Sr. were on a trip to Africa to call attention to the need to address the AIDS epidemic. In Abuja, Nigeria, he was asked to give a sermon on HIV/AIDS in the presidential chapel. This is that sermon/address.

JEFFREY SACHS and SONIA EHRLICH SACHS

Economists

AIDS and Africa: Where is the U.S.?

February 4, 2002

The sight was shocking. Peering into the medical ward of Queen Elizabeth Hospital was like peering into a corner of hell. AIDS has overtaken the hospital. Seventy percent of the medical-ward admissions are AIDS-related, but the hospital lacks the proper medications to treat the sick. So the patients come to die in ever increasing numbers, far beyond any capacity to manage. Two to a bed; sometimes three to a bed. When the beds overflow, the next wave of the dying huddle on the floor under the beds, to stay out of the way of families, nurses, and doctors passing through the wards. The constant low-level moans and fixed gazes of emaciated faces fill the ward.

These patients are dying of poverty as much as they are dying of AIDS. In the next corridor is an outpatient service that offers AIDS drugs. Four hundred or so patients are successfully being treated with antiretrovirals. They are the tiny fraction who can afford to pay approximately $1.00 per day out of pocket for the medicines.

The treatment has been successful. CIPLA, the Indian generics producer, supplies the drugs; the patients take them twice a day; and they get better. No great complexity, no unusual complications of toxicity, no struggles to achieve patient adherence to the drug regimen. Just a doctor prescribing medicines, and his patients responding.

A few miles away, one sees the implications of the dying fields that Africa has become. A village in Malawi is like a giant orphanage, in which a few elderly and wizened grandmothers look after the children of their dead and dying sons and daughters.

Enter a village and suddenly one is surrounded by dozens of children, a handful of elderly, and almost nobody of working age. On the day of our visit, it turns out, the few remaining men are off to a funeral. The grandmothers talk softly of their lost children as their orphaned grandchildren squat quietly nearby.

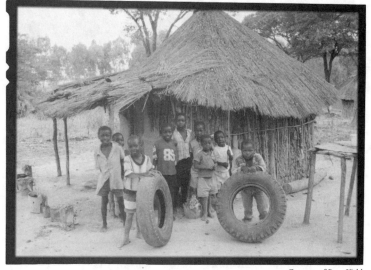

Courtesy of Pam Kidd

One grandmother shows us the rotting, bug-infested millet that she will use to make the gruel that keeps her and her wards barely alive. A beautiful young girl proudly tells us that she is in the second grade. She walks barefoot three kilometers early each morning to get to school. She wants to go to college, says her grandma. To make it, she will have to beat forbidding odds.

The rich world is an accomplice to the mass deaths in Africa. Why aren't U.S. leaders visiting the hospitals, villages, and health ministries in Africa to ensure that the United States is doing all it can do to stop the deaths? Why aren't U.S. leaders talking to African doctors? We are spending tens of billions of dollars to fight a war on terrorism that tragically claimed a few thousand American lives. Yet we are spending perhaps one- one hundredth of that in a war against AIDS that kills more than five thousand Africans each day.

A report of the Commission on Macroeconomics and Health of the World Health Organization shows that a tiny share of rich-country income—one penny of every $10.00 of GNP—would translate into eight million lives saved each year in the poor countries.

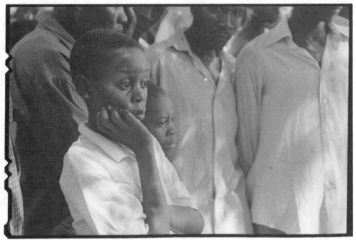

Courtesy of World Vision

The rich world is running out of excuses. Every misconception we've heard about treating AIDS patients—that the drugs don't work in Africa, the patients wouldn't adhere to "complex" regimens, that the doctors aren't qualified or can't be trained—has been matched by similarly lazy misconceptions about foreign assistance.

We've been told that any aid would be wasted, that debt relief would be squandered by corruption. We've been told that it's not "cost effective" to spend a tiny fraction of our own income to save millions each year, as if it's cost effective to let a generation die, to allow the collapse of Africa's tottering health care system, and to stand by as tens of millions of children are orphaned.

Debt-relief foes in Congress have warned that the benefits of debt cancellation would never reach the poor. We found the opposite. In each country that we visited on this trip—Malawi, Uganda, Ghana— the government is pursuing a meticulous and transparent process to ensure that budgetary savings from debt relief are actually channeled into urgent social sectors. The problem is not waste or corruption; the problem is that the extent of help from the United States and Europe is so meager in the face of the enormous crisis.

In a small room in Uganda, the intermingling of beauty and unnecessary suffering touched us more deeply than we could have imagined. A singing troupe of HIV-infected individuals, all likely to die in the next few years for lack of access to life-saving meds, sang to us with great power, charm, and bravery of their struggles.

Rock star Bono, traveling with our group, reached for his guitar. With haunting beauty, he responded with his magnificent ballad "I Still Haven't Found What I'm Looking For." The Ugandans swayed rhythmically to his pure and gripping tones. The tears flowed freely.

The U.S. complicity in Africa's mass suffering, unless reversed, will stain our country. Africa is the place where we will confront our own humanity, our morality, our purposes as individuals and as a country.

Reprinted by permission of Jeffrey Sachs.
From The Boston Globe, *2002.*

KEVIN MAX

Recording Artist

Twenty-First Century Miracle Man

The face of Christ is not the face of prosperity. It is not the face of comfort or of the church. The sharp lines and haunted eyes are of sorrow, the brow of hope and the chin of confidence. The face of Christ

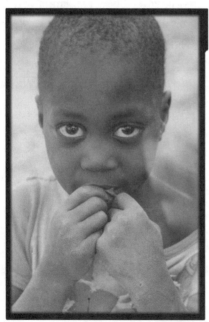

Courtesy of World Vision

knows poverty and is familiar with rejection, ignorance, and hatred. When I think of a picture of a modern Jesus, a 21st century miracle man, my internal eye sees these things. My inner-mind portrait would be of a man, undernourished yet strong. He would be full of compassion, magic, and mystery, a rebel with a cause. This portrait would involve the controversial settings of his social agenda. Instead of well-dressed, comfortable, fattened faces, he would be surrounded by lepers, prostitutes, and men of low stature. The destitute knew him and called him *friend*. The common sinner felt the brush of his hand and the power of his love. The leper, thief, and demon-possessed knew his name, not by circumstance but by relationship.

The face of Christ is the face of utter, shameless love and grace. It is a temple of acceptance, a warm skull of familiarity. When I think of a 21st century Jesus, I see a friend to the AIDS victim, a person of humility and understanding. If I had to search for him, I would start in the streets and alleyways of the restless.

I would find him in the mists of Africa.

I would find him seeking me.

When I think of all the ignorance and hatred in the world, all of the injustice, I think of the Nazarene strung up on a cross. "No man can come to the Father, but through *me*," he said time and time again. I have to believe this same Jesus opens his arms time and time again to the orphans and victims of AIDS. I am like you, I live in a comfortable home, drive a nice car and watch movies from a DVD player. In fact, I found out about the AIDS in Africa crisis, not through the Church, but from the lips of a rock 'n roll star. I am guilty of living well, and in comfort, and hiding within the shadows of our majestic American steeples. I would hope we could walk out of our comfort, once in a while, to feel the heat of Truth on our faces.

With the falling of the two towers and the rising of hatred in the Middle East, there are many opportunities for prayer. I have felt the need to see the plight of Africa with my own eyes, but for a time will do what I can through prayer and intercession. This is something we all can do, something we were made to do. We can effect culture and we can make a difference: flesh and blood were made for soul work.

The face of Christ is not the face of prosperity; it is the face of giving.

JESSE HELMS

United States Senator

We Cannot Turn Away
March 24, 2002

This year, more than half a million babies in the developing world will contract from their mothers the virus that causes AIDS, despite the fact that drugs and therapies exist that could virtually eliminate mother-to-child transmission of the killer disease.

It is my intent to offer an amendment with Senator Bill Frist of Tennessee to the Emergency Supplemental Appropriations bill to add $500 million—contingent on dollar-for-dollar contributions from the private sector—to the U.S. Agency for International Development's programs to fight the HIV/AIDS pandemic. The goal of this new money will be to make treatment available for every HIV-positive pregnant woman. As President Bush would say, we will leave no child behind. There is no reason why we cannot eliminate, or nearly eliminate, mother-to-child transmission of HIV/AIDS—just as polio was virtually eliminated forty years ago. Drugs and therapies are already provided to many in Africa and other afflicted areas. Only more resources are needed to expand this most humanitarian of projects.

The stakes could not be higher. Already in many African nations, an entire generation has been lost to AIDS. Mother-to-child transmission of HIV could eliminate another. Although reliable numbers are hard to come by, experts believe that more than two million pregnant women in sub-Saharan Africa have HIV. Of these, nearly one-third will pass the virus onto their babies through labor, child-birth, or breast-feeding, making mother-to-child transmission of AIDS the number one killer of children under ten in the world.

There will be obstacles to achieving universal availability of drugs and therapies. Many African nations lack the infrastructure and trained personnel to deliver health care on this scale. Some governments may not be cooperative. My amendment will provide the administration with the flexibility to deliver the necessary assistance while addressing these obstacles. For instance, if the new Global Fund to Fight AIDS, Tuberculosis and Malaria is deemed the most efficient way to deliver assistance, then the President can transfer money there.

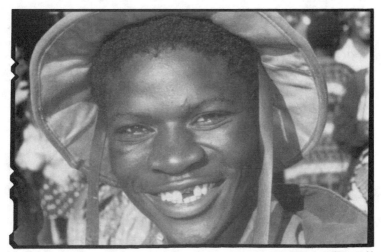

Courtesy of Pam Kidd

The United Nations has already set an ambitious goal of reducing the portion of infants infected with HIV by 20 percent in 2005 and by 50 percent in 2010. We can accelerate these goals, saving hundreds of thousands of lives, with a larger investment of public and private funds now. Private contributions, either financial or in kind—such as the donations of the drug nevirapine by the German pharmaceutical company Boehringer Ingelheim—are an essential part of a successful anti-AIDS strategy.

In addition, national commitment is absolutely essential. The

Government of Uganda can serve as an example. Through the leadership of Uganda's First Lady, Janet Museveni, that country has cut in half its HIV infection rate.

In February, I said publicly that I was ashamed that I had not done more concerning the world's AIDS pandemic. I told this to a conference organized by Samaritan's Purse, the finest humanitarian organization I know of. Indeed, it is their example of hope and caring for the world's most unfortunate that has inspired action by so many. Samaritan's Purse is led by Franklin Graham, son of Billy Graham—both of whom I count as dearest friends—but the organization was founded by the late Bob Pierce. Dr. Pierce's mission was to "Let my heart be broken with the things that break the heart of God." I know of no more heartbreaking tragedy in the world today than the loss of so many young people to a virus that could be stopped if we simply provided more resources.

Now, some may say that, despite the urgent humanitarian nature of the AIDS pandemic, this initiative is not consistent with some of my earlier positions. Indeed, I have always been an advocate of a very limited government, particularly as it concerns overseas commitments. Thomas Jefferson once wrote eloquently of a belief to which I still subscribe today: that "our wisdom will grow with our power, and teach us, that the less we use our power the greater it will be."

The United States has become, economically and militarily, the world's greatest power. I hope that we have also become the world's wisest power, and that our wisdom will show us how to use that power in the most judicious manner possible, as we have a responsibility to those on this earth to exercise great restraint.

But not all laws are of this earth. We also have a higher calling, and in the end our conscience is answerable to God. Perhaps, in my eighty-first year, I am too mindful of soon meeting Him, but I know that, like the Samaritan traveling from Jerusalem to Jericho, we cannot turn away when we see our fellow man in need.

Reprinted by permission of
The Office of Senator Jesse Helms.

KOFI ANNAN

Secretary-General of the United Nations

We Can Beat AIDS
June 25, 2001

The world cannot underestimate the threat of AIDS, but it would be equally wrong to fall into despair. The facts about AIDS are stark: twenty-two million people have died, with last year's total of three million the highest yet. In some African countries a quarter of the population is infected with HIV, the work force is shrinking and decades of progress in raising living standards is being wiped out. The same will soon happen to countries elsewhere—in Asia, Eastern Europe, the Caribbean—unless they take drastic action now. And no country is immune. But in the last few months the world has awakened at last, not only to the scope of the problem, but to the reality that we are not powerless against it.

The special United Nations session on AIDS that opens today comes at a time when we have more reason for hope than we have had in the last twenty years. Even poor and middle-income countries can protect themselves by combining prevention and treatment, as Brazil, Senegal, and Thailand have shown. Even the worst affected countries can confront the disease and contain its spread, as Uganda has shown. International drug companies have slashed the prices of antiretroviral drugs and other AIDS-related medicines in the poorest countries. And in Africa, political leaders have faced up to the problem as never before.

Two months ago, at the African summit in Abuja, Nigeria, I

sensed a new spirit of urgency. All the nations represented there undertook to increase the share of resources they devote to health, and to AIDS and HIV in particular.

The proper strategy has also become clear: prevention of new infection, above all by teaching young people how to avoid it and by providing the medicines that can prevent transmission from mother to child; care and treatment for those infected, for humane reasons but also to bring people in for testing, which they are likely to avoid when there is no hope of treatment; more research toward vaccines and a cure; and finally, protection of those whom AIDS has left most vulnerable—starting with children it has orphaned.

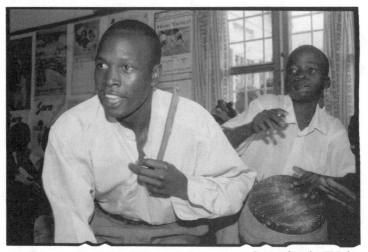

Courtesy of Jonathan W. Rodgers

These are achievable objectives. All this can be done, in the whole of the developing world, for an annual expenditure of $7 billion to $10 billion. That is five times what is now being spent—and it would need to be sustained for many years—but it is only a quarter of New York City's budget. The world can surely find this amount.

Some of this money will have to be spent on improving general health care systems in poorer countries to equip them to provide for the effective treatment of AIDS.

Some of the money will come from within the poorer countries most affected by AIDS, but I believe the public in the richer nations is also ready to contribute significantly. It is in these nations' self-interest as well as humanitarian interest to do so, since no country can be unaffected by a global disaster of this magnitude.

Governments, foundations, commercial companies, private individuals—all have been coming forward in the past few months, wanting to play their part in the global effort. Some already know how they want to spend their money and to whom they should give it. Others want to contribute to a global fund that can make sure the right strategy is followed and simplify the application procedures for countries that need assistance. At this week's special session of the United Nations General Assembly, I am sure more countries will announce contributions.

Every day lost is a day when ten thousand more people become infected with HIV. We can beat this disease, and we must.

Reprinted by permission of Kofi Annan.
Originally published in The New York Times,
June 25, 2001.

OUT OF EDEN

Recording Artists

The First to Help

Our desire to be involved in the AIDS crisis stems from our African roots. Our families are from South Africa, so we have always had a heart for its people. We have experienced firsthand the devastation that has been going on there. Something must be done. We must be proactive.

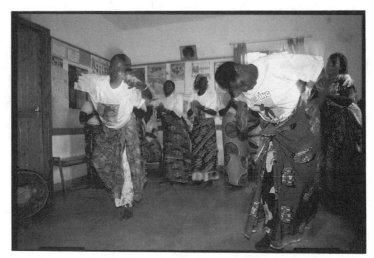

Courtesy of Jonathan W. Rodgers

Recently, we partnered with World Vision, an organization with a heart for the AIDS crisis, to sponsor one hundred African kids at our concerts. At $26 per month per child, we have had a great response. We have also teamed up with the DATA organization. We have encouraged people to get involved by signing petitions at our concerts—petitions that go to Congress to ask that they vote to drop Africa's debt and add money to the budget to support the AIDS crisis. We want people to continue adding their names to these petitions. We want them to write to their congressmen. We aren't always able to take money out of our pockets, but our government can.

The biggest responsibility, however, lies not with the government, but with the believers of the world. I appeal to all Christians who read this to live as Jesus lived, walk as Jesus walked. The Bible tells us that Jesus instructed his disciples to love their neighbors and give to the poor. He urged believers who professed his name to help those less fortunate than themselves. Yet, over time, Christians have put these things aside. We have forgotten what the Bible says. We have not done our job in loving our neighbors. We, as believers, need to abandon our hypocrisy and set the example. We must be the first to help those in need.

Written for The aWAKE Project,
Copyright © 2002 by Andrea Baca.

DIKEMBE MUTOMBO

Professional Athlete, NBA
UNDP Youth Emissary

Corporate Council on Africa: Remarks
September 5, 2000

My name is Dikembe Mutombo, and as you may know, I was born in the Democratic Republic of the Congo (formerly Zaire). This past July, I had the honor of attending the XIII International Conference on AIDS that was held in Durban, South Africa. I was invited to attend the event as the Youth Emissary on behalf of the United Nations Development Programme.

My function as the Youth Emissary was to encourage young people to act responsibly and recognize the devastating impact that HIV/AIDS is having on their lives and communities. A recent UN report states that in countries such as South Africa and Zimbabwe, where a fifth or a quarter of the adult population is now infected, AIDS is set to claim the lives of around one-half of all fifteen year olds. If this pandemic is not brought under control, half of all fifteen year olds in sub-Saharan African will not make it to age thirty. For example, when I visited the Goodwin's Clinic in Durban, I was saddened to see how many young Africans were living with the AIDS virus. This was something I have never experienced before in my life. It is becoming more sorrowful each time I visit Africa during the off-season, performing at free basketball clinics where up to two thousand children a day show up. I get a first-hand opportunity to witness the most catastrophic health crisis in the world and the toll that it is taking on my continent and on the young future generations.

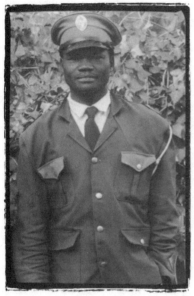

Courtesy of Pam Kidd

As you know, the health and development of a country is closely linked to the health of its people. Children of the world are in a state of crisis. They are our richest natural resource and caring for them is an investment in the truest sense of the world. We ignore their development at our own peril. It is through them that we invest in the future of the economy, in the future security of the world, and in its future social health and stability.

I didn't go to South Africa because it's the worst place in the world, I went there because AIDS is taking away the future of my continent, and AIDS is everybody's problem.

Thank you for your attention and God bless.

Reprinted by permission of The Dikembe Mutombo Foundation.

LUCI SWINDOLL

Author and Speaker

Love Brings Healing

One of the most meaningful Saturdays I ever spent was April 7, 2000. A group of us from Women of Faith were in Chennai, India, getting acquainted with World Vision's work.

At the Chennai Integrated HIV/AIDS Care Center we met a dozen beautifully dressed women—all of whom had HIV or AIDS. Most were in their twenties or thirties. Greeting us was Dr. Punitha, the thirty-four-year-old Indian psychiatrist who was the leader of this facility. She had a warm smile as she told us, "The women could hardly sleep last night. They were so excited about your visit today. They've planned testimonies and dances for you and have been practicing for weeks."

The World Vision-supported center provides counseling, advice, health education, treatment of minor ailments in slum communities, and a temporary home for women with no place to live.

One of the women, Lakshmi, gave her testimony about how she came to the center. Her husband had died of AIDS after twenty years of marriage, leaving her and three of their five children infected. Dr. Punitha was notified of this woman's inability to move to the treatment center because of her emaciated condition. She was living with her parents, who had isolated her in their home because of their fear of the AIDS contagion.

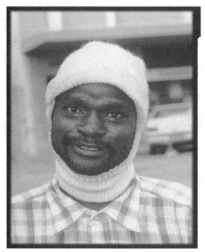
Courtesy of Pam Kidd

Dr. Punitha had Lakshmi hospitalized and later moved to the care center. The other women received Lakshmi and her children with love that seemed to know no bounds. In time, Lakshmi grew stronger. Her dancing reflected her joy in being alive and her appreciation for having a place to live with her family.

That day at the HIV/AIDS center is a very rich memory in my mind. It was wonderful and moving to see for myself the fine work that was being done for so many by so few.

Would that the Christian churches of America would answer that same call. We, as believers in Jesus Christ, are lights in darkness; therefore we must carry the torch. Although AIDS is an international tragedy of epic proportions, we serve a mighty God who grants courage and wisdom in fighting the good fight of faith. Let's step out of the shadows and lead others into battle.

Reprinted by permission of World Vision.

MICHAEL TAIT

Recording Artist

The Effect of AIDS on the Conscience, Heart and Mind

I would imagine that to most people AIDS seems very distant, very hard to understand. If it hasn't affected someone close to us, we feel naively immune to the disease. When my sister, Sharon, contracted the disease, it took her a long time before she told anyone. I imag-

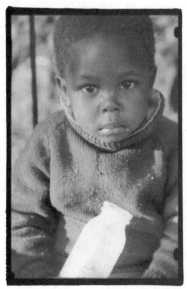
Courtesy of Pam Kidd

ine she felt shame and fear at our response. Actually, I think she might have told my girlfriend first. That was early in 1995; in June of 1996 she passed away.

I never really gave much thought to AIDS—it hadn't become personal to me yet. That all changed when Sharon told us she had HIV and it had progressed to full-blown AIDS. That was hard—it triggered all sorts of fears in me. I remember thinking to myself, *if I kissed her, would I get it? What if she starts bleeding, should I help her?*

70

Should I wear gloves? If I somehow got her saliva on me, would the disease spread to me? Because I didn't know enough about AIDS, fear was my first reaction. I remember feeling almost like Sharon had become a leper. When AIDS touches your family, it changes your perspective. It changed our family. It changed my life.

When she passed, she left two beautiful girls behind. It was and still is very difficult. You don't get over the effect of AIDS. You move beyond, and hopefully come out on the other side with the determination to do your part to help end this disease. As Michael Tait, brother and uncle, I need to find my individual part. As part of the Church, I need to share our story and help the Church take an active part in reaching out to those affected. If you haven't been affected personally—you are blessed. That does not mean you have the privilege to ignore the heartbreak that this has brought to those around the world. Africa is in an extreme situation. We need to be concerned and have compassion for those people. We need to find a way as the Body of Christ to be involved.

People who have this disease need our love more than ever. Don't run from people with AIDS. We need to fight the fear to ostracize them because of the disease. We need to love these people as Christ loves these people. Christ loved and reached out to the Samaritan woman at the well—she was very different than him. We need to ask for His love to reach out to the suffering and comfort them in what may be their last days on earth.

Written for The aWAKE Project,
Copyright © 2002 by Michael Tait.

CHARLIE PEACOCK

Recording Artist

Africa, It's Personal

It was the 4th of July, Independence Day—the first for the United States since 9/11. I took a seat at the desk in the recording studio, reached up and turned the television on to CNN. I'd come in to retrieve my journal for a little morning writing and while closeby, surrendered to the temptation to check my email. Glancing at the television, I could see the President speaking from a podium, framed by veterans of war, fleshy symbols of freedom's fight. I looked down at my laptop where two messages had popped up, both urgent.

The first was in regard to friend and colleague Grant Cunningham who'd fallen and suffered a head injury while playing soccer. The message urged all who received it to "please pray." I shut off CNN and immediately began talking to God about what I trusted was a matter of mutual concern—our friend Grant. Next, I printed out the email to give to my wife Andi, so that she would talk with God about it as well.

The second email was in regards to the ongoing and urgent crisis in Africa, specifically poverty and the deadly AIDS virus. Though the first email might have appeared to be more personal, the second was no less.

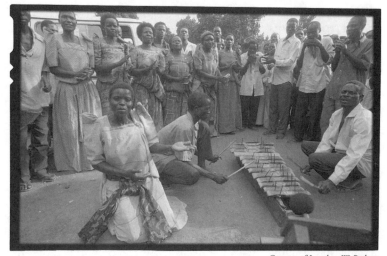

Courtesy of Jonathan W. Rodgers

As a student-follower of Jesus and the ways of God, I'm committed to having my understanding of *personal* undergo a lifelong, incremental transformation. What's personal to God is step-by-step becoming personal to me as well. This is as it should be, given that God gave stewardship of his personal creativity to the human family.

The email regarding Africa contained a link to an article on the Christian music community's involvement with U2's Bono and an organization called DATA, a dual acronym for stopping the crises of Debt, AIDS, and Trade in Africa, in return for Democracy, Accountability, and Transparency in Africa. Several people in our Nashville tribe (and beyond) have gathered together to help DATA tell the story of Africa's brokeness and need. The email updated me on our progress and pointed me to a second link, an interview with Bono on the subject of DATA and Africa, in which he assured the interviewer that the world would be hearing from the sleeping giant that is the church.

I believed him (and still do). I wanted to shout "Amen!" and cue Al Green for a chorus or two. Judging by his actions in recent years, one could surmise that Bono has been doing a lot of talking with God about matters of mutual concern. He has been taking things like the care of widows and orphans very personally, as anyone should who claims to stumble after Jesus. The Book of James reminds readers that the religion God accepts as pure and good is the care of orphans and widows in their distress (like those in Africa), and keeping oneself from being polluted by the world's ways of being and doing (like caring less about your comfortable western lifestyle and more about your dying neighbor across the ocean).

The usually cranky prophet Jeremiah tied one's knowledge of God to this very idea when he spoke of the good King Josiah: "'He defended the cause of the poor and needy, and so all went well. Is that not what it means to know me?' declares the Lord."

Yet it's not just the poor and needy widows and orphans of Africa that have Bono speaking like the preacher of a congregation you'd actually like to join. I'm also quite sure this DATA idea is more than a pontificating rock star's grand gesture. From where I stand it looks to me like real care and concern for the creativity of God overall—widows and orphans included, or especially. He's championing the summation of the Jewish law—love of God and neighbor—as well as the care-taking role given to the human family in the beginning. If you take all of life personally, as Jesus did, then the shape and territory of love expands farther than you or I can imagine. Nevertheless, most of us can find Africa on the map.

Bono's passion for Africa (God's creativity in need of love and care), has bumped into us here in Music City. The collision woke more than a few sleepy musicians, myself included. Everyday more and more music folk are being urged by the Spirit to tell the story of Africa and the story of the only good response, the God response. The one where the image of God in humankind, made alive by the breath of God, cares for what God loves, his creation. It's the response where men and women act congruent with the way they're made, and as a result actually look like what they are—God's direct representatives here on earth.

The wind of the Spirit is moving through the air. People are tuning into the right channels. You can hear the very personal problem of Africa cutting through the distortion and racket of *me* and *mine*. The light is opening sleepy eyes. Distant concerns are coming near. Willing hearts and hands are bringing them even closer. Africa—God's creativity, filled with people made in his image, poor and needy.

Here's the action point: Talk to God and to each other about this important matter of mutual concern. Tell the story and let people know through word and deed that you are taking it personally. This is the way of Jesus.

Written for The aWAKE Project.
Copyright © 2002 by Charlie Peacock.

OLUSEGUN OBASANJO

President of Nigeria

Letter to the Southern Baptist Convention
August 15, 2000

M r. Adrian Rogers
Chairman
Southern Baptist Convention

Dear Mr. Rogers,

I write to you as a fellow believer, as a Baptist and one who tries through faith and practice to follow God's word in my role as democratically elected leader of Nigeria, a nation of 120 million people.

Before I was elected President last year, in the first democratic election in twenty years, I was chairman of Transparency International, a global anti-corruption foundation and in the 1990s, a member of the Commonwealth Eminent Persons Group that helped to broker the peaceful transition in South Africa. I was head of the military government that handed over power to a democratically elected government in 1979 and a keen farmer.

I write to you in a spirit of fellowship at the dawn of a new millennium, about the condition of my country and people and to ask you to remember us in your prayers, as well as in your practical testimonies to your Congressmen, who collectively have the power to lessen our suffering through forgiveness of our intolerable debt.

Presently, we are obliged to divert $1.5 billion of our meager resources to service our debts to Western creditors.

I lead a country that is at a critical stage in its transition to democracy, which I believe is the only path that will bring prosperity and peace to my people. We are a desperately poor country facing many formidable challenges. We also suffer from the unfair misunderstanding that we are a rich oil country that does not need debt relief. In spite of our oil endowment, our debt to export ratio is 250 percent, which both the IMF and World Bank agree is far too high for a developing country.

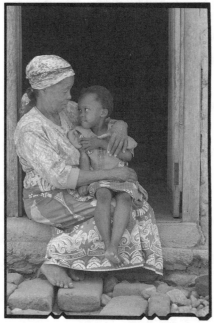

Courtesy of World Vision

The average per capita income for my fellow citizens is a paltry $300, as against an average of $29,240 for the United States. In 1979, we spent $2.25 per capita on education. In the same year the U.S. spent $1,546 for each person. Under our current budget, my government has been able to allocate only $3.00 per person to health. The U.S. government spends $4,080 on each citizen. These are the only resources we have to fight the threatened HIV/AIDS epidemic which accounts for about a million deaths annually and Malaria which is responsible for one in five of all childhood deaths in Africa.

Fellow Baptists, as you can see, the health challenge is pressing and I feel particularly passionate about this. But I can only spend $3.00 on each of our 120 million citizens, which scarcely covers for the cost of a mosquito net!

Like many of you in the Southern Baptist Convention, I am a

man of the book and never embarrassed to draw inspiration and wisdom from biblical authority. A verse that never fails to enlighten my thoughts is Leviticus, Chapter 25, which evokes the "'Ram's Horn Blast' to declare liberty throughout the land." I know that this biblical idea of Jubilee is also close to the hearts of all Americans, as it is the biblical text engraved on the side of the Liberty Bell in Philadelphia. It is the idea that the imposition of suffering upon the poor is an offence to God's holiness that drives our magnificent Baptist vision, particularly in the developing world.

The year 2000 is a jubilee year, which should restore the earth as in the concept of the Sabbath and promote friendship amongst all of its citizens. It is also a time for forgiveness. "You shall count off seven weeks of seven years, seven time seven years, so that the period forty nine years and you shall hallow the fiftieth year, and you shall proclaim liberty throughout the land to all its inhabitants" (Leviticus 25:8, 10).

My people cannot hallow the fiftieth year. And we enter a new millennium, not in a spirit of new beginnings but a millstone of debt grinds our country and its people into endless poverty. Nigeria borrowed $5 billion from Western creditors in 1978. Since then, we have paid back $16 billion. It may also surprise you to know that we still owe $31 billion! This is largely due to compound interest and interest rate fluctuation. Prophet Isaiah rallied against this form of economics when he chastised the creditors, "You add house-to-house and field-to-field until there is room for no one but you" (Isaiah 5:8). Jesus appealed to the creditors to be "merciful, as your father also is merciful" (Luke 6:34).

Fellow Baptists, we live in a world in which mankind is accumu-lating the greatest riches in all of its recorded history, yet I am writing to you almost in despair. I have just returned from a meeting with the leaders of the G8 in Tokyo, Japan, as representative of the G77 group of countries. I pleaded with the richest countries to give a billion people in the developing world a cause for celebration, at the dawn of this new millennium by canceling their unpayable debts. I left very disappointed.

Dear brothers and sisters in Christ, you have the power and influence, in your Congress to right this wrong. You can persuade your Congressmen and women to give millions of our citizens relief from the millstone of their debts—by writing the debts off the books. I know that if you take up the cause for debt cancellation in this jubilee year, you will not be alone. Millions of Christians all over the world support this. In the U.S. Congress, I was heartened to read about the moving testimony of one brother, Kasich, who called on the U.S. government to agree to debt cancellation this year "as a historic act of grace." Senior economists like Professor Jeffrey Sachs of the Harvard Business School have also supported the case.

So, fellow brothers and sisters in Christ, my call to you is not from the wilderness. There are many voices supporting our call. But we need your support too. Let us stand together in the great spirit of our Lord, in His mercy and forgiveness.

Thank you and God bless.
OLUSEGUN OBASANJO

Reprinted by permission of Adrian Rogers.

BONO

Recording Artist

Transcript of Video Message Recorded for Christian Music Festivals, plus Extrapolations

Thanks for listening to this video message—I really appreciate it. I went to Africa recently and came back with some facts I'd like to share with you. Some of you may know these, some of you may not, but they are all still mind-blowing.

Twenty-five million people in Africa now have HIV. Think about

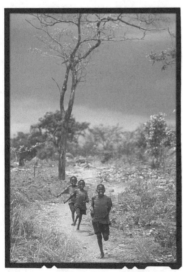

Courtesy of World Vision

that—twenty-five million people in Africa are HIV positive. Thirteen million children are orphans because their parents have died from AIDS—and this figure is expected to double by the end of the decade.

Today—in the next twenty-four hours—5,500 Africans will die of AIDS. Today in childbirth 1,400 African mothers will pass on HIV to their newborns.

If this isn't an emergency, what is? In the Scriptures we are not *advised* to love our neighbor, we are *commanded.* The Church needs to lead the way here, not drag its heels. The government needs guidance. We discuss; we debate; we put our hands in our pockets. We are generous even.

But, I tell you, God is not looking for alms; God is looking for action. He is not just looking for our loose change—he's looking for a tighter contract between us and our neighbor.

Africa is America's neighbor. Africa is Europe's neighbor. We are daily standing by while millions of people die for the stupidest reason of all: money.

There is a growing movement for Jubilee in the United States. I love that word Jubilee—it suggests joy in a new beginning free from the bondage of slavery of any kind. In this instance, economic slavery. Let's not forget that redemption is an economic term. We need to drop the debt and end the ridiculous situation where today's generations in the poorest countries have to spend what little they have paying back old loans rather than investing in health, education, and clean water. We need to make trade rules more fair. If we're serious, we need to let these countries put their products on our shelves and stop refusing them what we demand for ourselves—autonomy in managing their own markets.

And finally, all rich countries need to increase development assistance to fight AIDS and poverty in Africa. This is not about throwing money away but about using our national wealth to improve the lives of the poorest people in the world. At the moment, of the twenty-two richest countries, the U.S. is at the bottom of the list when you look at how much the government is planning to give to foreign assistance as a proportion of overall wealth: 0.15 percent of GDP. And almost half of this goes to middle income countries. The UK and Ireland are at 0.32 percent. All countries need to get the level of the Scandinavians: 0.7 percent. Americans are generous people. This doesn't make sense. Their personal giving is in line with everyone else.

I should be preaching to the converted here. There are 2,300 verses of Scripture pertaining to the poor. History will judge us on how we deal with this crisis. God will judge us even harder.

Let me tell you about Jonah. In Soweto, I met a man called Jonah. He was an extraordinary-looking young man, striking and fit. Five years ago he weighed half his body weight; he was covered in scars from scratching a terrible skin rash; he was bed-ridden with TB. He had no hope—the cost of medication was totally beyond his family's reach. But, he managed to get onto a Medicine sans Frontiers program, and soon his life was transformed by anti-retrovirals. We were excited; he was excited. He told us that his wife had died of AIDS, leaving him with their two children. His kids made him feel even more glad to be alive and healthy. We were excited again. Then he told us that his new love was also HIV positive. She is not part of the ARV program, and there is no way she can afford the drugs.

So here was Jonah's dilemma. He said he could share his drugs with her and risk that they have no effect. Or, he could give his drugs to her knowing that his children would lose their father to AIDS. Or he said, *I can keep the drugs and lose the woman I love, now the mother to my children.* In my opinion, that's a decision that no civilized world should ask Jonah to make.

Look, sometimes we've just got to do what we're told. The children of God have to listen to their Father in Heaven. It's easy to think that Africa's problems are caused by natural calamity and corruption and have nothing to do with us. That's part of the problem, but the truth is also that the relationship between the developed and the developing world has been so wrong so for long—corrupt actually.

It's the start of the twenty-first century; it's time to put this right. Charity alone will not work. We need a new partnership based on justice and equality. We need to remind ourselves that God will not accept our acceptance of lives made wretched by a geographical accident of latitude and longitude.

We must wake up the sleeping giant of the Church; we must set alarm clocks to rouse our politicians who also slumber. The choice is there before each and every one of us: to stop and tend to the distant pilgrim sick on the side of the road, or, a nervous glance, and we turn away . . . away from the pilgrim, away from God's grace.

Written for The aWAKE Project,
Copyright © 2002 by Bono.

PART TWO

Knowledge

NADINE GORDIMER

Writer, Winner of the 1991 Nobel Prize in Literature, UNDP Goodwill Ambassador

Once Upon a Time

Someone has written to ask me to contribute to an anthology of stories for children. I reply that I don't write children's stories; and he writes back that at a recent congress/book fair/seminar a certain novelist said every writer ought to write at least one story for children. I think of sending a postcard saying I don't accept that I 'ought' to write anything.

And then last night I woke up—or rather was wakened without knowing what had roused me.

A voice in the echo-chamber of the subconscious.

A sound.

A creaking of the kind made by the weight carried by one foot after another along a wooden floor. I listened. I felt the apertures of my ears distend with concentration. Again: the creaking. I was waiting for it; waiting to hear if it indicated that feet were moving from room to room, coming up the passage—to my door. I have no burglar bars, no gun under the pillow, but I have the same fears as people who do take these precautions, and my windowpanes are thin as rime, could shatter like a wineglass. A woman was murdered (how to they put it) in broad daylight in a house two blocks away, last year, and the fierce dogs who guarded an old widower and his collection

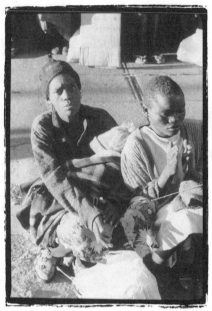

Courtesy of Pam Kidd

of antique clocks were strangled before he was knifed by a casual labourer he had dismissed without pay.

I was staring at the door, making it out in my mind rather than seeing it, in the dark. I lay quite still—a victim already—but the arrhythmia of my heart was fleeing, knocking this way and that against its body-cage. How finely tuned the senses are, just out of rest, sleep! I could never listen intently as that in the distractions of the day; I was reading every faintest sound, identifying and classifying its possible threat.

But I learned that I was to be neither threatened nor spared. There was no human weight pressing on the boards, the creaking was a buckling, an epicentre of stress. I was in it. The house that surrounds me while I sleep is built on undermined ground; far beneath my bed, the floor, the house's foundations, the stopes and passages of gold mines have hollowed the rock, and when some face trembles, detaches and falls, three thousand feet below, the whole house shifts slightly, bringing uneasy strain to the balance and counterbalance of brick, cement, wood and glass that hold it as a structure around me. The misbeats of my heart tailed off like the last muffled flourishes on one of the wooden xylophones made by the Chopi and Tsonga migrant miners who might have been down there, under me in the earth at that moment. The stope where the fall was could have been disused, dripping water from its ruptured veins; or men might now be interred there in the most profound of tombs.

I couldn't find a position in which my mind would let go of my body—release me to sleep again. So I began to tell myself a story; a bedtime story.

In a house, in a suburb, in a city, there were a man and his wife who loved each other very much and were living happily ever after. They had a little boy, and they loved him very much. They had a cat and a dog that the little boy loved very much. They had a car and a caravan trailer for holidays, and a swimming-pool which was fenced so that the little boy and his playmates would not fall in and drown. They had a housemaid who was absolutely trustworthy and an itinerant gardener who was highly recommended by the neighbours. For when they began to live happily ever after they were warned, by that wise old witch, the husband's mother, not to take on anyone off the street. They were inscribed in a medical benefit society, their pet dog was licensed, they were insured against fire, flood damage and theft, and subscribed to the local Neighbourhood Watch, which supplied them with a plaque for their gates lettered YOU HAVE BEEN WARNED over the silhouette of a would-be intruder. He was masked; it could not be said if he was black or white, and therefore proved the property owner was no racist.

It was not possible to insure the house, the swimming pool or the car against riot damage. There were riots, but these were outside the city, where people of another colour were quartered. These people were not allowed into the suburb except as reliable housemaids or gardeners, so there was nothing to fear, the husband told the wife. Yet she was afraid that some day such people might come up the street and tear off the plaque YOU HAVE BEEN WARNED and open the gates and stream in...Nonsense, my dear, said the husband, there are police and soldiers and tear-gas and guns to keep them away. But to please her –for he loved her very much and buses were being burned, cars stoned, and schoolchildren shot by the police in those quarters out of sight and hearing of the suburb—he had electronically-controlled gates fitted. Anyone who pulled off the sign YOU HAVE BEEN WARNED and tried to open the gates would have to announce his intentions by pressing a button and speaking into a receiver relayed to the house. The little boy was fascinated by the device and used it as a walkie-talkie in cops and robbers play with his small friends.

The riots were suppressed, but there were many burglaries in the suburb and somebody's trusted housemaid was tied up and shut in a cupboard by thieves while she was in charge of her employers' house. The trusted housemaid of the man and wife and little boy was so upset by this misfortune befalling a friend left, as she herself often was, with the responsibility for the possessions of the man and his wife and the little boy that she implored her employers to have burglar bars attached to the doors and windows of the house, and an alarm system installed. The wife said, She is right, let us take heed of her advice. So from every window and door in the house where they were living happily ever after they now saw the trees and sky through bars, and when the little boy's pet cat tried to climb in by the fanlight to keep him company in his little bed at night, as it customarily had done, it set off the alarm keening through the house.

The alarm was often answered—it seemed—by other burglar alarms, in other houses, that had been triggered by pet cats or nibbling mice. The alarms called to one another across the gardens in shrills and bleats and wails that everyone soon became accustomed to, so that the din roused the inhabitants of the suburb no more than the croak of frogs and musical grating of cicadas' legs. Under cover of the electronic harpies' discourse intruders sawed the iron bars and broke into homes, taking away hi-fi equipment, television sets, cassette players, cameras and radios, jewellery and clothing, and sometimes were hungry enough to devour everything in the refrigerator or paused audaciously to drink the whisky in the cabinets or patio bars. Insurance companies paid no compensation for single malt, a loss made keener by the property owner's knowledge that the thieves wouldn't even have been able to appreciate what it was they were drinking.

Then the time came when many of the people who were not trusted housemaids and gardeners hung about the suburb because they were unemployed. Some importuned for a job: weeding or painting a roof; anything, *baas*, madam. But the man and his wife remembered the warning about taking on anyone off the street. Some drank liquor and fouled the street with discarded bottles. Some begged, waiting for the man or his wife to drive the car out of the electronically-operated gates. They sat about with their feet in the gutters, under the jacaranda trees that made a green tunnel of the street—for it was a beautiful suburb, spoilt only by their presence—and sometimes they fell asleep lying right before the gates in the midday sun. The wife could never see anyone go hungry. She sent the trusted house-maid out with bread and tea,

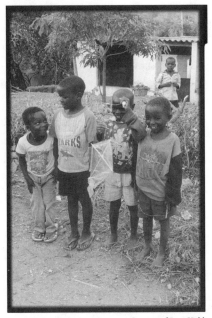

Courtesy of Pam Kidd

but the trusted housemaid said these were loafers and *tsotsis*, who would come and tie her up and shut her in a cupboard. The husband said, She's right. Take heed of her advice. You only encourage them with your bread and tea. They are looking for their chance…And he brought the little boy's tricycle from the garden into the house every night, because if the house was surely secure, once locked and with the alarm set, someone might still be able to climb over the wall or the electronically-closed gates into the garden.

You are right, said the wife, then the wall should be higher. And the wise old witch, the husband's mother, paid for the extra bricks as her Christmas present to her son and his wife—the little boy got a Space Man outfit and a book of fairy tales.

But every week there were more reports of intrusion: in broad daylight and the dead of night, in the early hours of the morning, and even in the lovely summer twilight—a certain family was at dinner while the bedrooms were being ransacked upstairs. The man and his wife, talking of the latest armed robbery in the suburb, were distracted by the sight of the little boy's pet cat effortlessly arriving over the seven-foot wall, descending first with a rapid bracing of extended forepaws down on the sheer vertical surface, and then a graceful launch, landing with swishing tail within the property. The white-washed wall was marked with the cat's comings and goings; and on the street side of the wall there were larger red-earth smudges that could have been made by the kind of broken running shoes, seen on the feet of the unemployed loiterers, that had no innocent destination.

When the man and wife and little boy took the pet dog for its walk round the neighbourhood streets they no longer paused to admire this show of roses or that perfect lawn; these were hidden behind an array of different varieties of security fences, walls and devices. The man, wife, little boy and dog passed a remarkable choice: there was the lowcost option of pieces of broken glass embedded in cement along the top of walls, there were iron grilles ending in lance-points, there were attempts at reconciling the aesthetics of prison architecture with the Spanish Villa style (spikes painted pink) and with the plaster urns of neo-classical facades (twelve-inch pikes finned like zigzags of lightning and painted pure white). Some walls had a small board affixed, giving the name and telephone number of the firm responsible for the installation of the devices. While the little boy and the pet dog raced ahead, the husband and wife found themselves comparing the possible effectiveness of each style against its appearance; and after several weeks when they paused before this barricade or that without needing to speak, both came out with the conclusion that only one was worth considering. It was the ugliest but the most honest in its suggestion of the pure concentration-camp style, no frills, all evident efficacy. Placed the length of walls, it consisted of a continuous coil of still and shining metal serrated into jagged blades, so that there would be no way of climbing over it and no way through its tunnel without getting entangled in its fangs. There would be no way out, only a struggle getting bloodier and bloodier, a deeper and sharper hooking and tearing of flesh. The wife shuddered to look at it. You're right, said the husband, anyone would think twice . . . And they took heed of the advice on a small board fixed to the wall: Consult DRAGON'S TEETH The People For Total Security.

Next day a gang of workmen came and stretched the razor-bladed coils all round the walls of the house where the husband and wife and little boy and pet dog and cat were living happily ever after. The sunlight flashed and slashed, off the serrations, the cornice of razor thorns encircled the home, shining. The husband said, Never mind. It will weather. The wife said, You're wrong. They guarantee it's rust-proof. And she waited until the little boy had run off to play before she said, I hope the cat will take heed...The husband said, Don't worry, my dear, cats always look before they leap. And it was true that from that day on the cat slept in the little boy's bed and kept to the garden, never risking a try at breaching security.

One evening, the mother read the little boy to sleep with a fairy story from the book the wise old witch had given him at Christmas. Next day he pretended to be the Prince who braves the terrible thicket of thorns to enter the palace and kiss the Sleeping Beauty back to life: he dragged a ladder to the wall, the shining coiled tunnel was just wide enough for his little body to creep in, and with the first fixing of its razor-teeth in his knees and hands and head he screamed and struggled deeper into its tangle. The trusted housemaid and the itinerant gardener, whose 'day' it was, came running, the first to see and to scream with him, and the itinerant gardener tore his hands trying to get at the little boy. Then the man and his wife burst wildly into the garden and for some reason (the cat, probably) the alarm set up wailing against the screams while the bleeding mass of the little boy was hacked out of the security coil with saws, wire-cutters, choppers, and they carried it—the man, the wife, the hysterical trusted housemaid and the weeping gardener—into the house.

PHILIP YANCEY

Author

Jogging Past the AIDS Clinic

Some of my best "reading" time occurs as I jog along Chicago's lakefront, outfitted with Walkman and headphones, listening to books recorded on cassette tape. One winter the city's dingy streets and rat-gray skies formed a perfect backdrop for the book I had selected: Daniel Defoe's *A Journal of the Plague Year*. In meticulous, matter-of-fact prose he describes the bubonic plague that afflicted London in 1665.

In the account (which renders history in the form of realistic fiction), Defoe wanders the streets of a ghost city. Over 200,000 people have fled London, and those who remain barricade themselves indoors, terrified of human contact. On main thoroughfares, where steady streams of people once trod, new grass grows. "Sorrow and sadness sat upon every face," says Defoe. At the peak of the plague, 1500 to 1700 people died each day, their bodies collected nightly for burial in cavernous open pits. The book describes gruesome scenes: dead children locked in the permanent grip of their parents' rigor mortis, live babies sucking in vain at the breasts of just-dead mothers.

As I listened, Defoe's account took on particular poignancy in view of a modern-day plague. My wife and I live in a neighborhood populated by many gays and not a few drug users. I could not avoid

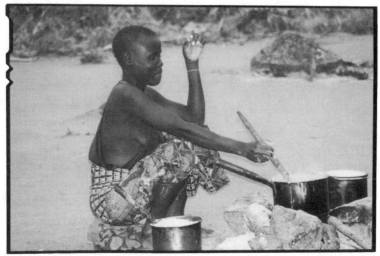

Courtesy of Pam Kidd

reflecting on the parallels between Defoe's time and our own as I jogged past a clinic for AIDS patients and dodged lampposts plastered with "AIDS Benefit" posters. Compared with the Great Plague, the AIDS epidemic has afflicted a much smaller proportion of the population, but it has stirred up a remarkably similar response of hysteria.

In Defoe's day, it seemed that God's molten wrath was being poured out on the entire planet. Two bright comets appeared in the sky each night—sure signs, said some, of God's hand behind the plague. Wild-eyed prophets roamed the streets, one echoing Jonah with his cry, "Yet forty days and London shall be destroyed!" Another walked around naked, balancing a pan of burning charcoal on his head to symbolize God's judgment. Still another naked prophet dolefully repeated the same phrase all day long: "Oh, the great and dreadful God! Oh, the great and dreadful God. . . ."

We have our modern version of these prophets. Most are well clothed, however, and they tend to narrow the focal point of God's judgment down to one particular group, the homosexuals, who are disproportionately represented among AIDS sufferers in the U.S. In some circles I can almost detect a sigh of relief, a satisfaction that at last "they are getting what they deserve." Former Surgeon General C. Everett Koop, and evangelical Christian, received boxes full of hate mail whenever he dared to suggest otherwise.

The AIDS crisis taps into a mysterious yearning among human beings, a deep-rooted desire that suffering ought to be tied to behavior. I have a book on my shelf, *Theories of Illness,* that surveys 139 tribal groups from around the world; all but four of them perceive illness as a sign of God's (or the gods') disapproval. The author notes that the few who doubt such doctrine probably changed their beliefs after prolonged contact with modern civilization.

Virtually alone among all civilizations in history, our modern, secular one questions whether God plays a direct role in such human events as plagues and natural catastrophes. (Even we have our doubts: insurance policies specify certain "acts of God.") We are confused. Did God single out one town in the Southeast to be leveled by a tornado, as a message of judgment? Does he withhold rains from Africa as a sign of his displeasure? No one knows for sure. But AIDS—ah, there's a different story. Beyond dispute, the likelihood of AIDS transmission increases among those who engage in promiscuous sex, or share dirty needles.

For some Christians, AIDS seems to satisfy at last the longing for a precise connection between behavior and suffering-as-punishment. In a general sense, the connection has been established—in the same way that smoking increases risk of cancer, obesity increases risk of heart disease, and heterosexual promiscuity increases risk of venereal disease. The natural consequences of such behavior include, in many cases, physical suffering; scientists recognize this fact and advertise it widely. But the lurking question remains: Did God send AIDS as a specific, targeted punishment?

Other Christians are not so sure. They see a grave danger in playing God, or even interpreting history on his behalf. Like Job's friends, we can too easily come across as cranky or smug, not prophetic. "Vengeance is mine," God said, and whenever we mortals try to appropriate his vengeance, we tread on dangerous ground. Judgment without love makes enemies, not converts. Among the gays in my neighborhood, Christians' statements about the AIDS crisis have done little to encourage reconciliation.

Even the apparent cause-and-effect tie to behavior in AIDS raises troubling questions. What of "innocent" sufferers, such as the babies born to infected mothers or those who received the virus in a blood transfusion? Are they tokens of God's judgment? And if a cure is suddenly found—will that signify and end to God's punishment? Theologians in Europe expostulated for *four centuries* about God's message in The Great Plague; but it took only a little rat poison to silence all those anguished questions.

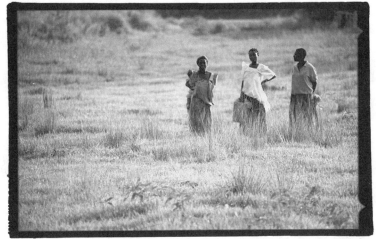

Courtesy of Jonathan W. Rodgers

Reflecting on these two plagues, the scourge of the buboes that killed off a third of humanity and the modern scourge with its kindred hysteria, I find myself turning to an incident from Jesus' life recorded in Luke 13:1-5. When some people asked him about a contemporary tragedy, here is how he responded:

> Do you think that these Galileans were worse sinners than all the other Galileans because they suffered this way? I tell you, no! But unless you repent, you too will all perish. Or those eighteen who died when the tower in Siloam fell on them—do you think they were

more guilty than all the others living in Jerusalem? I tell you, no! But unless you repent, you too will all perish.

Then Jesus followed up with a parable about God's restraining mercy. He seems to imply that we "bystanders" of catastrophe have as much to learn from the event as do the sufferers themselves. What should a plague teach us? Humility, for one thing. And gratitude that God has so far withheld the judgment all of us deserve. And compassion, the compassion that Jesus displayed to all who mourn and suffer. Finally, catastrophe joins together victim and bystander in a common call to repentance, by abruptly reminding us of the brevity of life. It warns us to make ourselves ready in case we are the next victim of a falling tower—or an AIDS virus.

I have yet to find any support in the Bible for an attitude of smugness: *Ah, they deserve their punishment; watch them squirm.* Indeed, the message of a plague seems directed to survivors as much as to the afflicted. I guess AIDS holds as much meaning for those of us who jog past the clinics as for those who suffer inside.

Reprinted by permission of Eerdmans Publishing Group.
From Philip Yancey, I Was Just Wondering, *rev. ed.,*
© 1989, 1998 Wm. B. Eerdmans Publishing Company,
Grand Rapids, MI. Used by permission.

JAMILA PAKSIMA

Journalist

A Day in South Africa
November 9, 2001
Pienaar, South Africa

Deep in the heart of this land, at the far ends of the shadows that still fall from the days of apartheid, is hope for a righteous future for South Africa's children. But the promise of shared humanity, equal access, education, and health care is still a dream in the making—the new South Africa is seven years young. Those who work as warriors and architects of this new democracy say, "You must be patient; transition takes time." But these new years of freedom have been hard and increasingly violent. Some say they are getting harder especially for young children. Here, the quest for freedom and progress is too often derailed by disease, poverty, and distrust. Today truth is revealed quickly, but denial and resignation are squashed with the demands for real change. With nothing but courage as armor, women and children and young girls in the new South Africa are now speaking out . . . and the truth of their pain deserves the world's attention.

Life here is still about struggle. For the young girls of this country the hope of a childhood paved with innocence, joy, and purity is tragically disappearing into tales fit for fables of days past. In the province of Mpumalanga, which in Zulu means "the place of the rising sun," every twenty-six seconds a woman or girl child is raped.

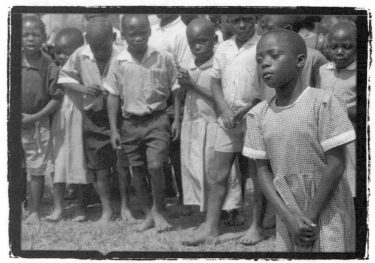

Courtesy of Jonathan W. Rodgers

South Africa boasts the highest rape statistics in the world. One in five South Africans between the ages of fifteen and forty-nine is HIV positive. This means rape victims face a long and painful death sentence.

Experts tell me here rape is fueled by anger, poverty, and ignorance; many blame the rise on "the myth." The myth is explaining the unexplainable: "sex with a virgin child will cure a man of AIDS." In villages across South Africa and provinces like Mpumalanga infant rape, child rape, and gang rapes are daily occurrences. Nine years old, two years old, nine months old . . . I cannot comprehend the numbers I see on Excel spreadsheets that Barbara Kenyon, founder of the grassroots organization Greater Nelspruit Rape Intervention Project (GRIP) shares with me. These images of soul-stealing acts are unimaginable, but this is why I am here working on a documentary in South Africa. Kenyon shows me and anyone else who will listen what she calls *her proof.* Hoping her highlighted charts will raise funds, or the purchase of expensive HIV prevention anti-retroviral medication, and raise attention to the needs of raped children in her community.

I need to see more than these charts.

Barbara Kenyon suggests I go to the village of Pienaar where violence is spreading the HIV venom to the innocent children playing on streets. This is Mary's street.

In the car with me is Fickele Sibiya, a twenty-four year old social worker with GRIP, and Nicky Lazar, my field producer. We sat in our rented car and watched life reveal itself here as we waited for school to end for nine-year-old Mary. We have come to hear her story. Poverty, idle men strolling, women carrying a single loaf of bread, and a child struggling with a six pound cabbage stream past our parked car on this bumpy, dusty road. We stare; they stare. I am taken by the sight across the street—children left at home alone, busy and happy skipping rope cleverly made out of plastic grocery bags. Three doors down we can hear a large group of young men singing and drinking. It is 1:00 PM in the afternoon, and they are clearly drunk and probably unemployed. Fickele warns the children to run away if the men try to talk to them.

This is the new free South Africa, and every face I see here has a need. We sat on this road watching these children play and eat the carrots we shared with them. After two hours Fickele says, "There she is . . ."

I see Mary and her aunt walking towards us on the dusty street. Three months ago Mary was raped by her stepfather. Sweet, shy, quiet Mary.

She wanted to talk. I set up my camera.

He would force himself on her, cover her mouth tightly with his hand, and she never screamed.

"He did it on Monday, Tuesday, Wednesday, Thursday . . ." she remembered each time, but could not say the words "every night." Mary endured the violations for more than a week, but the physical pain finally forced her to tell. She told the truth to her mother with her step-father standing in the same room. For the truth, Mary was forced to watch him beat her mother. The women went to the police, and he pleaded for forgiveness and apologized. Mary and her mother stood their ground, and he was arrested and put in prison. No one told Mary's mother there was help for her daughter, maybe because the local government here is opposed to the efforts of GRIP. Now, with fear, Mary's mother, grandmother and aunt wait for justice. Fickele tells me they will wait for at least a year for their day in court. In South Africa just 7 percent of litigated rape cases result in a guilty conviction.

Because of her stepfather's twisted acts, Mary's life has been cut short, but no one in her family has courage to tell her, not even her mother. Because of the repeated rapes, a grown man tearing his way inside a child, Mary is now HIV positive. Her mother is just learning how to face her own truth and ruined marriage—she too is infected by him with "the virus." This is the courage of one family to share their story. It is also the shame of a nation that they say isn't doing enough to help them.

POSTSCRIPT

Mary and her mother had their blood tested by GRIP. If Mary had told her mother about the violation immediately, and if her mother had brought her to GRIP within seventy-two hours of the first rape, there is a strong chance Mary could have been saved from HIV with anti-retroviral therapy.

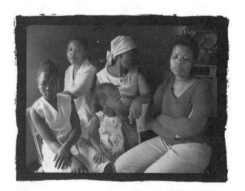

Courtesy of Jamila Paksima

I returned to South Africa June 2002 to continue filming my documentary on child rape in South Africa and went to the village of Pienaar in Mpumalanga to visit Mary and her mother. The news was terrible and tragically typical. An angry knock on the door in May was her stepfather. He had been let out of prison, and Mary's case against him had been dismissed. Pounding on the warped wooden door of their clay two room shack he shouted "he would kill them both . . . he wanted his clothes, and he wanted his Bible." The last thing Mary's mother heard about him was from a friend. The man whom she still calls the "rapist" is living with another woman and her daughter.

Written for The aWAKE Project.
Copyright © 2002 by Jamila Paksima.

STEPHEN LEWIS

Former Canadian Ambassador to the UN

On Topic with Stephen Lewis: AIDS in Africa
Summer 2002

AIDS is already the single greatest health crisis that has faced humankind," says international AIDS expert Stephen Lewis. "If it hasn't overtaken every comparable plague in the past, it will overtake it in the future."

Poverty's hold on Africa means that HIV/AIDS wipes out entire families much more quickly than in the United States. Already weakened by food shortages or poor nutrition, a lack of access to clean water, and without money for medicine, parents who contract HIV/AIDS have little hope of extending their lives long enough to care for their young children.

Stephen Lewis, special envoy to the United Nations for HIV/AIDS in Africa, discusses these complex issues in this interview with *World Vision Today*. Stephen is a passionate advocate for children. He served as deputy executive director of the United Nations Children's Fund (UNICEF) from 1995-1999. Throughout his long career as a humanitarian and diplomat, he has championed many causes around the world, particularly related to Africa and HIV/AIDS.

Today, Stephen works closely with African leaders to ensure progress on the objectives outlined at last year's African summit on HIV/AIDS in Abuja, Nigeria: to halt the epidemic's further spread, reduce mother-to-child HIV transmission, provide care and treatment, deliver scientific breakthroughs, and to protect the vulnerable—especially orphans.

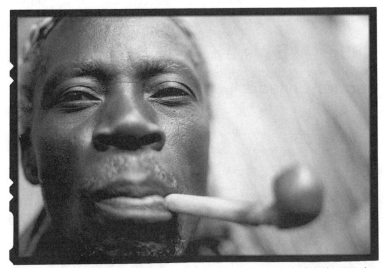

Courtesy of Jonathan W. Rodgers

We know that sub-Saharan Africa is currently the AIDS "hot zone." Why is the disease spreading so vigorously?

You have a combination of things: poverty, denial, stigma, gender oppression, transportation routes, migration, and civil conflict. The levels of poverty are so great that people's immune systems are tremendously fragile and susceptible to disease; there isn't the capacity to resist.

AIDS spread dramatically through heterosexual transmission in sub-Saharan Africa. Transportation routes moved truck drivers and others from one country to another, which allowed the pandemic to spread as travelers contracted HIV and carried it home. Conflict, too, is a vehicle for the spread of HIV/AIDS, through the sexual violence that occurs in refugee camps and among the internally displaced.

There is also terrible oppression of women who aren't able to refuse sexual contact, and with that the reality that sexuality is difficult to speak of. The stigma and denial are so intense that the pandemic can take root and spread rapidly, and no one will acknowledge and talk about it the way people talked about AIDS' spread through the homosexual and drug-using communities in the Western world. Put all these factors together, and it has been just a cauldron of self-immolation around the pandemic.

You say that culturally women can't refuse sex. Is that playing out in higher numbers of infected women?

Yes. In sub-Saharan Africa, women now constitute 55 percent of the infected, and the HIV/AIDS prevalence levels among women are regularly higher than men. In a number of communities in Botswana, the prevalence rate for women between 25 and 29 has reached 51.2 percent—one out of every two women in that age-range has effectively been served a death warrant.

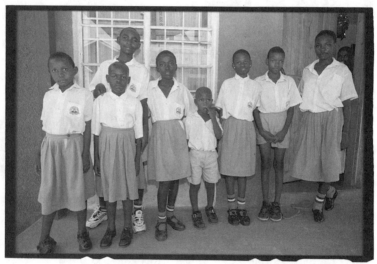

Courtesy of Jonathan W. Rodgers

How has AIDS affected families, communities, and entire nations in sub-Saharan Africa?

It has devastated family structures. Because mothers, fathers, uncles, and aunts are dead, grandmothers look after four, five, six,

10, 12 youngsters. There's an increasing phenomenon of child-headed households where [children] look after siblings with almost no shelter, no clothing, no food, and no money to pay for school. If ever there was a campaign needed in sub-Saharan Africa, it's to abolish school fees, because children who are orphaned by AIDS can't pay for tuition, books, or uniforms. They don't have a childhood left, let alone a family.

There isn't a sector of the social and economic infrastructure in these countries still intact. In the education sector, teachers are dying in large numbers, and students are removed from school to look after their ill parents. The health system is affected because there simply aren't the medical facilities to look after people; there aren't drugs to treat opportunistic infections, and there certainly aren't antiretroviral drugs [which work against the HIV infection] to treat full-blown AIDS. The agricultural sector is devastated because they can't till the land, they can't grow food, so people are hungry. President Olusegun Obasanjo [of Nigeria] said that parts of Africa are fighting against extinction. He's using apocalyptic language because in countries where the prevalence rate is more than 20 percent, you often feel as though you're standing in a graveyard.

If this is Africa's apocalypse, why isn't more being done for the suffering? Can we prolong a mother or father's life through antiretroviral drugs?

The drug companies have brought prices way down, but they're still out of reach of the vast majority of people afflicted with the disease. Of the 28 million people infected, only an estimated 30,000 to 50,000 are being treated. There is a tremendous effort to find the money to subsidize the cost or to provide the drugs free. Antiretrovirals are not the cure, but they can prolong life. Even more important, they actually encourage prevention, because if people have hope of life going on, they will get themselves tested.

What about behavior? Is it changing?

Sexual behavior is changing. Family Health International, which does a lot of work in Kenya, says that the decline in HIV infection rates is found largely in communities where prevention work is being done around [the topics of] abstinence, fidelity, condoms, early marriage, and multiple partners.

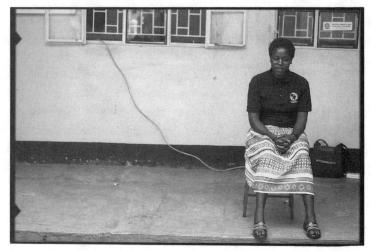

Courtesy of Jonathan W. Rodgers

What can nongovernmental organizations (NGOs) like World Vision do right now?

There is so much valuable and hopeful work at the community level. NGOs like World Vision that have a good reputation for doing things on the ground can form partnerships with these community-based organizations to provide care, prevention, orphan care, counseling. Another thing that has to be done by NGOs, including those in the faith-based community, is to speak out with alarm when they see delinquency—delinquency among governments where the pandemic is rampant, or in the response of the donor community. All voices have to be added to indict those who are moving too slowly, perpetuating denial, or refusing to get involved. The faith community has a big constituency; it cares deeply; and it knows that this thing can be defeated.

What's the most important thing Americans can do to respond to AIDS?

The most important thing is to become involved with an organization engaged in fighting the pandemic. Give them support when they put pressure on Congress or the president for more money. Support their work in the developing world. Give financially. Simply get involved, even if it's attending meetings, writing letters, making phone calls, stamping envelopes, sending e-mails. It's more important than giving a few dollars—it's actually embracing the issue as part of one's life, because there has never been an issue like AIDS. You simply can't write off an entire continent of between 600 and 700 million people.

Reprinted by permission of World Vision.

GEORGE W. BUSH

President of the United States of America

HIV/AIDS in Africa: Rose Garden Speech
June 19, 2002

Good morning. The global devastation of HIV/AIDS staggers the imagination and shocks the conscience. The disease has already killed over twenty million people, and it's poised to kill at least forty million more.

In Africa, the disease clouds the future of entire nations and threatens to hold back the hopes of an entire continent. In the hardest-hit countries of sub-Saharan Africa as much as one-third of the adult population is infected with HIV, and 10 percent or more of the schoolteachers will die of AIDS within five years.

The wasted human lives that lie behind these numbers are a call to action for every person on the planet and for every government. So, today, my administration is announcing another important new initiative in the fight against HIV/AIDS . . .

One of our best opportunities for progress against AIDS lies in preventing mothers from passing on the HIV virus to their children. Worldwide, close to two thousand babies are infected with HIV every day, during pregnancy, birth or through breast-feeding. Most of those infected will die before their fifth birthday. The ones who are not infected will grow up as orphans when their parents die of AIDS. New advances in medical treatment give us the ability to save many of these young lives. And we must, and we will.

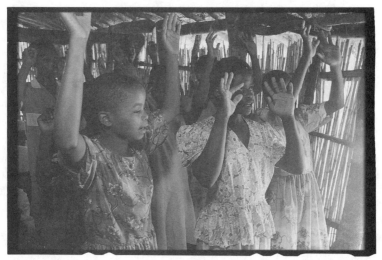

Courtesy of World Vision

Today I announce that my administration plans to make $500 million available to prevent mother-to-child transmission of HIV. This new effort, which will be funded during the next sixteen months, will allow us to treat one million women annually, and reduce mother-to-child transmission by 40 percent within five years or less in target countries.

I thank all the members of Congress who supported this initiative, especially Senators Frist and Helms. Their visionary leadership on this issue will mean the difference between life and death for hundreds of thousands of children.

Our initiative will focus on twelve countries in Africa and others in the Caribbean where the problem is most severe and where our help can make the greatest amount of difference. We'll pursue medical strategies that have a proven track record. We'll define specific goals. We will demand effective management. When the lives of babies and mothers are at stake, the only measure of compassion is real results.

We have a three-part strategy. First, in places with stronger health care systems, we will provide voluntary testing, prevention, counseling, and a comprehensive therapy of anti-retroviral medications for both mother and child, beginning before delivery, and continuing after delivery. This combination has proven extremely effective in preventing transmission of the HIV virus.

Second, in places with weaker health care systems, we'll provide testing and counseling, and we will support programs that administer a single dose of nevirapine to the mother at the time of delivery, and at least one dose to the infant shortly after birth. This therapy reduces the chances of infection by nearly 50 percent.

Third, and most importantly, we will make a major effort to improve the health care delivery systems in targeted countries. This will allow more women and babies to receive the comprehensive therapy. It will allow for better and longer treatment and care of all AIDS victims. And it will lead to better health care in general for all the country's citizens.

We'll help build better health care systems by pairing hospitals in America and hospitals in Africa, so that African hospitals can gain more expertise in administering effective AIDS programs. We'll also send volunteer medical professionals from the United States to assist and train their African counterparts. And we will recruit and pay African medical and graduate students to provide testing, treatment and care.

This major commitment of my government to prevent mother-to-child HIV transmission is the first of this scale by any government, anywhere. In time, we will gain valuable experience, improve treatment methods, and sharpen our training strategies. Health care systems in targeted countries will get better. And this will make even more progress possible. And as we see what works, we will make more funding available.

The United States already contributes approximately a billion dollars a year to international efforts to combat HIV/AIDS. In addition, we plan to spend more than $2.5 billion on research and development for new drugs and new treatments. We've committed $500 million to the Global Fund to Fight AIDS and other infectious diseases, and we stand ready to commit more as this fund demonstrates its success.

Today's initiative is not a substitute for any of these efforts. It is not a substitute for further U.S. contributions to the Global Fund. This initiative will complement those efforts, and it is an essential new step in our global struggle against AIDS.

Today, I call on other industrialized nations and international organizations to join this crucial effort to save children from disease and death. Medical science gives us the power to save these young lives. Conscience demands we do so.

Thank you very much.

This speech is in the public domain.

DANNY GLOVER

Actor, UNDP Goodwill Ambassador

HIV/AIDS and Africa's Poverty

My fight against HIV/AIDS is a personal one. I have a brother who is affected by the disease. As an artist, I also have had numerous friends and colleagues who have suffered from it and died. As a result, I have learned about its path of destruction through individuals into families and extending into communities, societies, and nations. I know about its obvious and not so obvious impact on those it leaves behind. It was for these reasons that I decided two years ago to focus a good portion of my work as UNDP's Goodwill Ambassador on building a global movement to fight HIV/AIDS wherever it surfaces and—particularly—in Africa, which has been hardest hit.

The statistics are staggering. More than 450 million people today live with HIV: nine out of ten are in developing countries; three-quarters of those afflicted live in sub-Saharan Africa. In Botswana, children born today can expect to live to thirty-six. That's about half as long as they would have been able to live in their country if AIDS did not exist. Thirteen million children have lost either a mother or father or both parents to the pandemic since its medical detection three decades ago.

Over the last two years, I have tried to learn as much as I can about various aspects of HIV/AIDS in order to be a better communicator to audiences worldwide that need to be awakened to the damage it inflicts, and how they can protect themselves. Part of my learning process has taken me to visit townships near Johannesburg and Durban, South Africa—the global epicenter of the epidemic at the time of the XIII International AIDS Conference in July 2000.

Along with UNDP Youth Emissary and Philadelphia 76er basketball star Dikembe Mutombo of the Democratic Republic of the Congo, and other AIDS activists from around the world, I visited the unmarked grave of Gugu Dlamini. She had been stoned to death by her neighbors for having stated publicly that she was living with AIDS. Afterwards, we went to visit her township. People of all ages were there to greet us. They lived in modest homes but shared what-

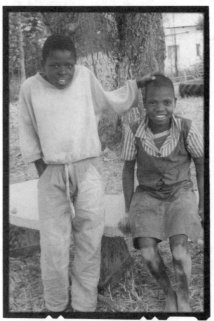

Courtesy of Pam Kidd

ever they had. Children and adults from the neighborhood came clustering around the front door of our host's home to watch the activities inside.

We were treated like kings, despite being surrounded by abject poverty. A local entertainment group showed us how they were getting information across to young people through pop songs and dances. As I listened to the messages they were conveying, and saw how hard people were trying to do it in such creative ways, I kept asking myself: *Why has Africa been hit so hard?*

There are some very obvious reasons. A disproportionate number of the world's poorest countries are in Africa. As a result, there is no money in them to build strong infrastructure to support adequate, well-distributed health care systems. Even if, for argument's sake, such infrastructure were in place, it would not be long before it would disintegrate due to lack of funding to maintain it.

Lack of money forces people to make unpleasant and sometimes self-destructive choices in order to survive. For instance, *Should I buy food for my wife and children or should I buy condoms? Given that I have an illness requiring antibiotics, should I use the available syringe that someone else has used, since I can't get a clean one because the hospital supply has been depleted for months? Should I, as a 13-year-old child, become a prostitute in order to be able to support my younger siblings after my parents have died of AIDS?*

There is a correlation between the extent of poverty and the HIV/AIDS epidemic in a given society. The poorer a community is, the higher the incidence of HIV/AIDS there. The Centers for Disease Control in the United States of America have documented this phenomenon, particularly among the African-American and Latino communities. That's why fighting HIV/AIDS requires a holistic approach that also addresses the issues of poverty. One dilemma feeds the other.

Reprinted by permission of UNDP.
From CHOICES magazine, September 2002.

RACHEL GBENYON-DIGGS

*Former Liberian Ambassador
to the United States of America*

Africa's Children: A Dying Breed

While the world's focus has been turned to the fight against terrorism and the crisis in the Middle East, a global security threat of potentially far greater consequences is gobbling up the lives and devouring the future of millions, in particular, Africa's children. In its Declaration of Commitment on HIV/AIDS, the UN General Assembly 2001 Special Session concluded that this wide-spread epidemic, "through its devastating scale and impact, constitutes a global emergency and one of the most formidable challenges to human life and dignity."[1]

More than forty million people in the world today live with HIV/AIDS; an estimated twenty-five million in sub-Saharan Africa alone. Some twelve million African children are orphaned by AIDS and abandoned. These poor, malnourished, uneducated, unvalued, and voiceless children represent a plague, tearing at the very economic and social fabric of the continent. Pertinent social indicators show the impact of HIV/AIDS on Africa's children is worse than a decade of war. And the epidemic has yet to peak!

How disturbing that a continent so rich in natural and human resources, that has given so many contributions to mankind, from the arts and sciences to religion, is now threatened with a future so bleak!

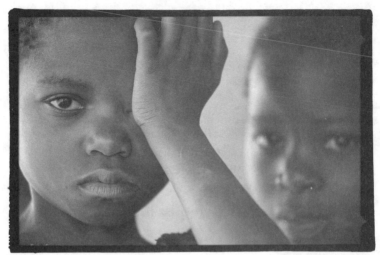

Courtesy of World Vision

Yet, the New Partnership for African Development, NEPAD, presented at the recent G-8 Summit in Calgary, with only a cursory mention of the HIV/AIDS pandemic, list a number of millennium development goals: an annual growth rate of 7 percent for fifteen years; fifty percent reduction in poverty by the year 2015; two-third reduction in infant mortality rates; reduction in maternal mortality rates by three-quarters; school eligibility for every child, thereby re-enforcing the principle of gender equality. But how can any responsible leadership envisage or plan a viable future for sub-Saharan Africa without putting the AIDS crisis at the heart of the analysis? It simply cannot! In addressing the issue of communicable diseases, in particular, HIV/AIDS, tuberculosis and malaria, the NEPAD text states categorically: "unless these epidemics are brought under control, real gains in human development will remain an impossible hope."[2] Africa's future—and that of the world—is inextricably linked to the defeat of the HIV/AIDS pandemic. With increasing trans-hemisphere movement of people and produce, no nation or continent is immune to the plague that finds its ground zero in another continent.

A recent study released by the United Nations Education and Social Council shows that four out of every ten primary school age children are now not in school in sub-Saharan Africa. It is not uncommon to see children pulled out of classrooms to look after ailing parents, many attempting to survive in child-headed households after the death of parents. And even if the children attend school, teachers are dying at an alarming rate. At the 2002 Children's Summit, organized by the UN, participants were stunned to learn that over the past year alone, a million African children lost their teachers to AIDS. The government of Mozambique estimates that seventeen percent of its teachers will die of AIDS by the end of this decade.

If not as graphic, this picture is as painful as the pictures of the atrocities perpetrated during the civil war in Sierra Leone. The world watched in horror as the media brought into our homes innocent children with their limbs chopped in acts so barbaric as to defy logic and human understanding. Will it take a repeat to wake up the world to this plague that has its epicenter in Africa?

Enlightened leadership that mobilizes and properly channels political will and money can defeat this global scourge. At the 2001 AIDS Summit held in Abuja, Nigeria, the Secretary-General of the United Nations formally proposed the Global Fund, and asked for $7 to $10 billion per year from all sources, but particularly from governments. The rich nations have contributed, thus far, $2.1 billion, but over three years, and no proposed schedule of payments from the contributing countries. At the higher and more realistic level of $10 billion, it then amounts to about 7 percent of the need over those three years. At the present rate of need to disburse the $2.1 billion in the coffers, the Global Fund will very soon run out of money. It has been suggested that the accepted formula applied to the budget of the UN and its peacekeeping operations should apply for the Global Fund. Enlightened leadership must now take that suggestion and turn it into applied policy.

It seems incongruous that despite its enormous wealth in mineral and natural resources (oil, diamonds, gold, copper, uranium, titanium, the world's largest deposits of chromium, gum arabica, rubber, timber) that Africa's growth is so frustratingly slow. Could the stunted development be attributed to global foreign policy toward and trade relations with Africa? The pricing of all commodities is outside of African control (fixed by the consumers of natural resources). The funding for Africa's development programs and projects is determined by international financial institutions, often with disregard for national needs and cultural differences.

How else can it be explained that a continent so rich cannot provide basic health care for its people? The estimated annual expenditure on health per person in Africa is estimated to be as low as $10 US. In the small West African state of Liberia infant mortality rate stands at 134 per every 1,000 live births and under-five mortality at 235 per every 1,000 live births. (The infant mortality rate in developed countries is around five to six per 1,000). Prior to a military takeover in 1980, The World Bank classified Liberia as a "middle-income oil importing country";[3] with a growth rate "roughly on par with the growth rates experienced by Japan and West Germany."[4] Liberia, which endured a devastating civil war from 1989 to 1996, is now classified among the ten most underdeveloped countries in the world!

And yet the major exports to Africa in these times are arms, ammunitions and military training, worth several billion dollars, to bolster support to corrupt regimes! Research shows that in 1998, Africa suffered eleven major armed conflicts, more than any other continent. Africa is now classified as the world's most war-torn region. In this decade alone, thirty-two African countries have experienced violent conflict, and many face continuing civil war or the looming threat of renewed fighting.

How then can African governments afford to provide the HIV anti-retroviral drugs which even in the United States cost on average $15,000 US per person per year? How then can African governments fight the international pharmaceutical companies that put profits before patients, with agreements such as Trade Related Intellectual Property Rights (TRIPS). TRIPS require signatories to the World Trade Organization to grant patent protection to pharmaceutical products for a minimum of twenty years.

If we conclude that the rampant spread of HIV/AIDS is inextricably linked to powerlessness and poverty, which in turn give birth to violence, isn't it time to take the moral high road in stemming this all-consuming disease?

The world has always looked to the United States for enlightened leadership in times of crises. The Marshall Plan is an important demonstration of America's bold leadership. The plan to revitalize Europe's economy ensured peace for future generations. As the worlds only super power, America must recognize the threat of the HIV/AIDS pandemic to its continued leadership role and security interests.

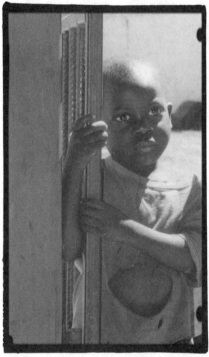
Courtesy of Pam Kidd

One of America's greatest thinkers, the late John Gardner, a scholar, ethicist and founder of Common Cause, put the case for America's responsibility to lead in clear and proper context. In his book *Excellence,* he reminded us that "the great advantage America gains from its widely dispersed leadership circles, has an offsetting cost."[5] Gardner was outraged that too often, "those who exercise power in [our] pluralistic society lack a sense of their role as leaders, a sense of the obligations which they have incurred as a result of the eminence they have achieved. . . . Or may well recognize their own leadership role with respect to their own special segment of the community but be unaware of their responsibility to the larger community."[6]

Millions of people around the world, living with the HIV/AIDS scourge, cannot help but wonder what is happening to America's sense of leadership and obligation. These are some of the same people who shed real tears when President Kennedy died because they truly felt they had lost one of their own. Let us turn back to Gardner: "If [Americans] are to recapture the sense of mission which our own survival demands, then our leaders must have the capacity and vision to call it out. In short, the varied leadership of our society must come to recognize that one of the great functions of leaders is to help a society to achieve the best that is in it."[7]

The HIV/AIDS pandemic cannot be relegated to the status of "Africa's problem." It is also America's crisis. The United States cannot abdicate its leadership role and accompanying responsibility. For in our truly global community, that which ravages the heart of Africa will, if left untreated, will in turn destroy the soul of America.

Written for The aWAKE Project.
Copyright © 2002 by Rachel Gbenyon-Diggs.

HELEN EPSTEIN and LINCOLN CHEN

Journalist and Scholar

Can AIDS Be Stopped?
March 14, 2002

During the past two decades, while virtually all Western countries experienced more or less constant economic growth, much of the rest of the world suffered a series of financial catastrophes—from the international debt crisis of 1982, to the Mexican peso crisis of 1994, to the Asian financial crisis of 1997, to the Russian default of 1998. The social consequences of these economic disasters—including impoverishment, mass unemployment, and ill health—have been felt almost entirely outside the West: in Africa, much of Asia, Latin America and the Caribbean, and the former Soviet Bloc.

While the causes of these crises were complex, much public criticism has been directed at some of the institutions that are attempting to establish rules for economic globalization—the World Trade Organization, the World Bank, and the International Monetary Fund. Protest movements have emerged, involving many different, sometimes conflicting, constituencies—from labor unions to environmentalists to college students to non-governmental organizations involved in health, social justice, and human rights. Their grievances more or less converge on a common theme: as Western governments, backed by multinational banks and corporations, push economic liberalization to extremes, they are exacerbating, and even exploiting, the vast social and economic inequalities that exist in the world.

Recently, George Soros, the financier and philanthropist, seems to have joined this chorus. In his new book *George Soros on Globalization*, Soros concludes that international finance and trade have outstripped the capacity of sovereign states to manage the politics of globalization.[1] Especially neglected has been the provision of global public goods, things needed by everyone but not produced by the marketplace, such as clean air and disease control. Instead of proposing to dismantle the WTO, the World Bank, and the IMF, Soros would like to see them strengthened, and complemented by stronger global institutions in social fields like health, such as the World Health Organization, and labor standards, such as the International Labor Organization. Successful globalization, he argues, requires effective global institutions devoted not only to finance and trade, but also to public health, human rights, environmental protection, and other public goods.

At the top of Soros's list of global social problems in need of attention is HIV/AIDS. Public concern over the global AIDS epidemic, particularly in Africa, has grown enormously in recent years, but there is considerable debate about what the international community can and should do about it. Especially controversial has been the high cost of antiretroviral drugs used to extend the lives of people with AIDS. The pharmaceutical companies that make these drugs price them beyond reach of the world's poor, but in November 2001 at the WTO meeting in Doha, Qatar, these companies were forced to accede to pressure from developing country governments, non-governmental organizations, and activists, and allow poor governments to adjust certain rigid patent rules applying to vaccines and drugs in order to protect public health. Despite this apparent triumph of international pressure, far more needs to be done. A coalition of governments and non-governmental organizations, led by the UN, recently launched the Global Fund Against AIDS, Tuberculosis, and Malaria (referred to here as the Global Fund), and its performance will test how well such a global institution can confront the most serious health crises of our time, and perhaps in all of human history.

1. To date, an estimated 50 million people have contracted HIV; about 25 million people in sub-Saharan Africa are infected, and about three million of these people die annually. In some countries, average life expectancy has fallen by more than a decade because of HIV/AIDS. Unfortunately, it has been only in the past two or three years that the gravity of the AIDS problem in Africa and other parts of the developing world has been fully recognized by those in the best position to do something about it, including many African presidents and prime ministers and such Western government leaders as Secretary of State Colin Powell, former President Bill Clinton, and the G8 heads of state at meetings in Okinawa and Genoa in 2000 and 2001.

Yet by 1985 many epidemiologists were already warning about the scale of the global AIDS epidemic.[2] Perhaps it should not surprise us that the AIDS crisis in Africa in particular has taken so long to become a matter of concern at such high political levels. In 1999, the UN Security Council declared AIDS in Africa an international security issue, because it further destabilizes already politically-fragile African nations. But how much does this really matter to the West, particularly the U.S.? The postwar history of the West's relationship with Africa suggests that when millions of Africans die, or when African states collapse, Western leaders often look away.

Diseases like malaria, respiratory infections, measles, and diarrhea, all preventable or curable and largely controlled in the West, continue to kill millions of African children, and yet U.S. overseas bilateral aid to Africa fell by half in the 1990s. During the cold war, the U.S. actively supported regimes in Liberia, Zaire, and South Africa that were responsible for the deaths of thousands more. The U.S. and Western Europe failed to intervene during the Rwandan genocide, and had it not been for a group of rock stars, Americans and Europeans might well have ignored the Ethiopian famine in the 1980s. Throughout the 1990s, U.S. funding for HIV prevention in developing countries averaged some $70 million per year, about the same as the U.S. military allocated for Viagra when this medication first became available.[3] Why did AIDS in Africa at last grab the rich world's attention? Why haven't similar deadly scourges of the third world done the same? One possibility is that when Western leaders, activists, corporation heads, and the general public look at the problems of the developing world, they mainly see reflections of problems in their own societies.

For many reasons, the suffering of African AIDS patients may draw international sympathy in a way that the suffering of malaria and diarrhea victims do not. For one thing, AIDS is a manifestly "global" disease; by the time it was first recognized in the early 1980s, HIV had already spread to nearly every continent. It has killed people of all races and classes, from the economically flourishing gay neighborhoods of San Francisco and New York to the poorest slums in Africa, Asia, Latin America, and the Caribbean.

Other infectious diseases were once as widespread and devastating as AIDS. Five hundred years ago, measles and smallpox introduced by Old World explorers and settlers decimated indigenous people in the New World. In 1918, "Spanish flu" killed millions around the world. Until the early twentieth century, malaria and typhoid claimed lives not only in the tropics, but also in Minnesota, England, and Arkhangelsk, Russia. During the past half-century, however, deaths caused by infectious diseases, particularly those common in childhood, became increasingly rare in industrialized countries. This led epidemiologists to associate certain patterns of disease with different stages of economic development. They classified communicable, nutritional, and reproductive problems such as malaria, tuberculosis, malnutrition, and death in childbirth as "diseases of poverty."

A second generation of diseases—which includes heart disease, stroke, diabetes, and cancer—were classified as "diseases of affluence," common in industrialized countries (although many people in developing countries, especially the well-to-do and middle class, also suffer from these chronic and degenerative diseases).

AIDS is part of a "third wave" of infectious, environmental, and behavioral pathologies that have accelerated in recent years. Some of these may be seen as "diseases of globalization" because they affect all countries and their ultimate control will require unprecedented global cooperation. During the past two decades, more than two dozen new infectious agents have been identified, including the prions that cause new variant Creutzfeldt-Jakob disease and the measles-like virus that killed fourteen horses and their trainer in Australia in 1994— along with new environmental health problems like global warming and ozone depletion. In addition, health problems associated with hazardous behavior, such as drug abuse, unsafe sex, traffic accidents, and violence, have also increased, particularly in societies undergoing rapid social change. The global distribution of these emerging diseases may explain why AIDS in particular is no longer seen as just another "third world" problem that people in the West feel they can largely ignore.

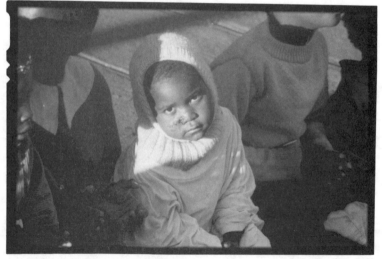

Courtesy of Pam Kidd

AIDS also raises troubling issues surrounding the global influence of private markets and the spread of infectious diseases. The collision between these two trends has created a kind of moral riptide with momentum of its own. Since 1996, HIV-positive patients in rich countries have had access to "cocktails" of drugs called antiretrovirals that can slow the progression of AIDS. These drugs are designed to attack the HIV virus, allowing the patient's immune system to repair itself and fight off opportunistic infections. Although the drugs do not cure AIDS, can have serious side effects, and do not work for all patients, their use has added many healthy years to the lives of thousands of people living with HIV in rich countries. There are now on the market around twenty antiretroviral drugs developed in the past fifteen years by pharmaceutical companies, the U.S. National Institutes of Health, and university laboratories.

Partly because they are so expensive, these life-saving drugs are largely inaccessible to the world's poor, especially the millions of HIV-positive people in Africa. One reason they are expensive is that international trade rules allow pharmaceutical companies a twenty-year patent, which effectively grants them a monopoly. During this time, the companies can charge whatever the market will bear. Until recently, patents on Western pharmaceuticals were valid only in a few countries, but that is now changing.

In 1994, Western governments concerned about protecting intellectual property pushed for an agreement on Trade-Related Aspects of Intellectual Property Rights (TRIPS) linked to membership in the World Trade Organization. TRIPS aims to extend patent protection to all WTO members, so that someone who produces a new CD or computer program, or invents a new pharmaceutical drug, will have the rights to that invention protected not only in the country in which it was first developed, but also in every country that joins the WTO. TRIPS was partly a response to the accelerated globalization of information which has made it easy for music and video pirates in China and generic drug makers in India, Thailand, and Brazil to copy Western inventions and products. Not all countries have signed on to TRIPS, but most have or will do so within the next decade.

Patenting drugs that could, if they were cheaply available, extend the lives and postpone the suffering of thousands or even millions of poor people in developing countries raises serious ethical concerns.

The development of antiretroviral drugs owes a great deal to gay HIV activists in rich countries, particularly in the U.S., who, beginning in the late 1980s, picketed the U.S. National Institutes of Health (NIH) demanding that more money be spent on AIDS research. They also demanded that the Food and Drug Administration accelerate the regulatory approval process for promising drugs. In the late 1990s, many of these same activist groups, including Act Up, began to ally themselves with campaigns led by such international development organizations as Médecins sans Frontières, Oxfam, and CARE. They claimed the pharmaceutical industry set exorbitant prices to enrich their shareholders while ignoring the plight of the world's poor. Why, they asked, were these life-saving drugs, now finally available, so expensive? Could they not be sold more cheaply to HIV-positive people in poor countries?

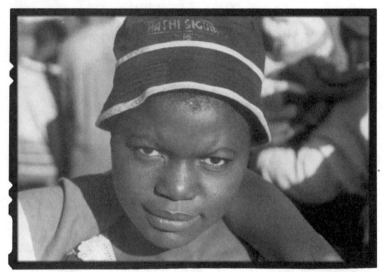

Courtesy of Pam Kidd

The debate over access to AIDS drugs in poor countries has taken place at the same time as an even larger debate about the mysteries of pharmaceutical pricing policies in general. There is some parallel between the AIDS drug debate and the debate over the high cost of prescription drugs for Americans, including Medicare patients. Drug companies are increasingly having to confront growing discontent among their customers in rich countries where they make most of their profits. These customers may be particularly sympathetic to poor Africans with AIDS because they share their concerns. Increasingly, Americans are asking: Why are drugs so expensive? How much profit is fair? Shouldn't moral standards apply to drug pricing for all people, poor Africans with AIDS as well as ourselves?

Concerns about the high cost of drugs in general have led to increased public scrutiny of the pharmaceutical industry, and this is beginning to pay off. Activists calling for greater use of generic drugs in poor countries with serious public health problems recently won a number of concessions. Generic drug companies in Brazil were already producing an antiretroviral cocktail before the country joined the WTO in 1996, and these drugs now form the basis of an exemplary treatment program, which offers free antiretrovirals to all Brazilians who need them. However it is not clear how easily Brazil's program could be reproduced in Africa, since Brazil's per capita income is ten times that of most African countries affected by AIDS, and only 0.5 percent of its

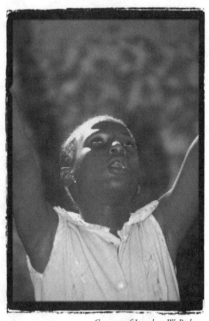

Courtesy of Jonathan W. Rodgers

citizens are HIV-positive, compared to between 5 and 35 percent in most countries of sub-Saharan Africa. The obstacles to distributing AIDS drugs in much of Africa are therefore much greater than they are in Brazil. Nevertheless, last April, the government of South Africa won a court case allowing it to manufacture its own generic versions of some patented drugs, and if Thabo Mbeki, South Africa's president, were to revise his idiosyncratic views on AIDS, a similar program could be launched there in the near future.[4]

At the recent WTO meeting in Doha, Qatar, poor governments were given permission to issue compulsory licenses, permitting local pharmaceutical manufacturers to produce generic versions of patented drugs for the local market in order to protect public health. Negotiations are underway to determine whether some countries might also be permitted to import patented drugs made by generic producers in other countries. In this way, a country such as Uganda that does not have the capacity to manufacture its own antiretrovirals might be permitted to purchase them from the Brazilian generics companies. To reduce the din of negative publicity, multinational pharmaceutical firms have been forced to offer AIDS drugs to a limited number of health institutions in developing countries at reduced prices under the Accelerated Access program, endorsed by the United Nations. However, this program offers only a limited number of drugs, and critics believe that only global generic competition will bring AIDS drug prices low enough so that they will reach a significant number of poor people in developing countries.

2. Indignation over the high cost of AIDS drugs has helped focus international attention on the global AIDS epidemic and by the end of 2001, an antiretroviral drug cocktail could be obtained in some developing countries for $300 to $500 per year, many times less than the price in the West. However, for a variety of reasons, including the sluggishness of government bureaucracies, the stinginess of drug companies, and the fact that even at these low prices the drugs are still too expensive and difficult to distribute, few AIDS patients in developing countries are actually receiving these drugs or, for that matter, any modern medications at all beyond the cheapest antibiotics. With this larger dilemma in mind, the UN recently launched the Global Fund for AIDS, Tuberculosis, and Malaria. But despite the fact that it is greatly needed and holds great promise, the Global Fund still faces great challenges. Kofi Annan originally proposed that between $7 and

$10 billion per year was needed, to be met by contributions from rich governments, corporations, and private donors. Thus far, however, the pledges total about $1.7 billion. Despite the rhetorical concern of Western donor governments, the commitments have been astonishingly stingy. The U.S. government has promised only $500 million over three years,[5] setting off a series of correspondingly disappointing commitments by other rich countries.

Difficult decisions will have to be made about how to allocate these limited resources to prevent and treat these three diseases. Opinions vary, for example, about how much of the Global Fund should go to pay for AIDS treatment. Last year, a group of Harvard academics proposed that some of the money be spent on buying discounted antiretrovirals from Western pharmaceutical firms. They cited various small-scale AIDS treatment programs including one based at the Clinique Bon Sauveur in Haiti and Médecins sans Frontières' Khayelitsha Project near Cape Town, South Africa, as evidence that administering antiretroviral drugs to poor AIDS patients in developing countries is feasible.[6] The greatest obstacle, say the directors of these programs, is the cost of antiretroviral drugs.

These small pilot projects are admirable and offer many practical lessons and hope, but there are grounds to question whether they could easily be extended throughout sub-Saharan Africa. Both the Bon Sauveur and Khayelitsha projects are currently administering antiretrovirals to only around one hundred patients each, while there are millions of people in Africa alone who might benefit from antiretrovirals. But experience shows that distributing even relatively simple drug regimens on such a large scale poses formidable obstacles. Programs in developing countries that aim to treat people with syphilis and tuberculosis, or even to distribute vitamin A supplements to children, show how difficult it is to deliver health care in such countries, even if the drugs are free or nearly so. An estimated 1.6 million women who give birth every year in those countries have syphilis, a disease that puts their newborns at high risk of deformity or death, even though the tests and drugs to treat it cost only about twenty-five cents. Hundreds of thousands of children go blind every year, and more than a million die, because they are deficient in Vitamin A. Vitamin A supplements, which need to be taken only twice a year, are virtually free. Of course some treatment and vaccination programs have been very successful, for example those for smallpox, polio, and onchocerciasis ("river blindness"), but vaccines for polio and smallpox need to be administered only a few times in a lifetime, while the oral dose to prevent the onset of onchocerciasis symptoms is taken once a year; and the recipients of such treatment, unlike AIDS patients, do not require ongoing care. And even these relatively simple programs have required enormous donor commitment and funding over long periods.

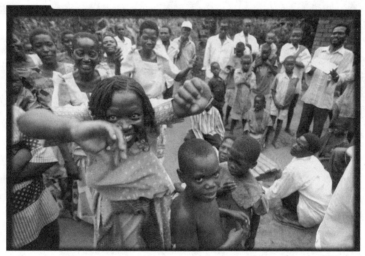

Courtesy of Jonathan W. Rodgers

The failure to deliver some even very cheap, simple treatments in developing countries is largely owing to the lack of sufficient trained and motivated health personnel, inadequate management and administrative capacity, and insufficient supplies of vehicles, refrigerators, lab reagents, and other basic equipment. For example, syphilis screening and treatment in antenatal care requires adequate staffing, an efficient referral system, reliable supplies of testing materials and drugs, an on-site rudimentary laboratory with quality control, and other resources that a great many health centers in poor countries simply do not have.

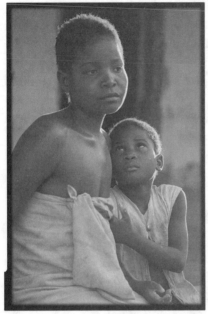

Courtesy of World Vision

Treating AIDS patients is far more complicated than testing for syphilis or administering Vitamin A drops. AIDS patients need counseling, laboratory tests, and ongoing clinical care to treat opportunistic infections and monitor drug side effects. Even if the drugs and other necessary supplies were available, and in most cases they aren't, antiretroviral treatment programs require considerable effort on the part of public sector health workers. But because of political instability, economic stagnation, and misguided health sector reform policies mandated by donor institutions such as the World Bank, the health workforce throughout sub-Saharan Africa has been collapsing. Doctors are severely underpaid, earning sometimes as little as $100 a month. Nurses and other staff earn far less. Low staff morale and moonlighting by government workers already severely undermine health services. During the past year, frustrated health workers in Zimbabwe and Uganda went on strike, and throughout sub-Saharan Africa trained doctors and nurses are leaving the public sector to seek better pay in the private sector, or migrating to other continents.

Any effective AIDS treatment program must endeavor to strengthen the health care system generally, especially the human infrastructure of front-line health workers, as well as meet the concerns of people affected by AIDS. The Harvard group proposed spending an additional $150 per year for the extra clinical work associated with each patient on antiretrovirals; but this may not be sufficient because adequately trained and motivated staff and organized health systems require many years of sustained investment. The antiretroviral treatment program at Clinique Bon Sauveur in Haiti, like many similar small-scale antiretroviral treatment programs in developing countries, is carried on through a health center that has long been well funded by foreign donors. Since Clinique Bon Sauveur was established fifteen years ago, it has always provided a far higher standard of care than is generally available in the public sector in Haiti, even before it began dispensing antiretroviral drugs to people with AIDS. Staff are paid regularly and decently, and know they have the resources, in drugs and supplies (in addition to antiretrovirals), to do their jobs well.

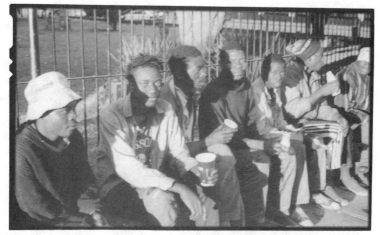

Courtesy of Pam Kidd

While antiretroviral drugs are important, they are not a panacea for the AIDS crisis in Africa. Indeed the debate over the high cost of the drugs has made AIDS in Africa appear to many to be merely a medical problem, when it is in fact far more than this. When an American or European becomes ill with AIDS, it is often mainly a matter for the patient and his doctor. Friends and family may grieve, but the effect of AIDS on an African family is of an entirely different order. This is because AIDS kills and weakens the adults who grow the food and earn the money that supports everyone else. The dependency ratio in Africa is much higher than it is in the West, not only because there are so many young children, but also because there are so many unemployed people, and most countries have no social safety net. Most sub-Saharan African workers are farmers, but because of inequitable land distribution and declining prices for Africa's agricultural products, farmers increasingly depend on relatives who are migrant workers or casual laborers in urban areas.

Migrant workers are particularly at risk of HIV, because of their youth and because of the loneliness and social anomie in the hostels and urban slums where many of them end up. When a South African mine worker, for example, becomes sick or dies of AIDS, he may leave behind in his rural home village as many as ten or twenty destitute

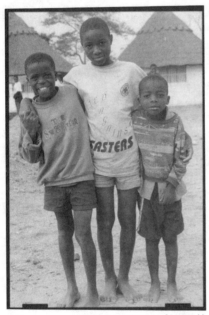

Courtesy of Pam Kidd

dependents, including children, wives, in-laws, brothers and sisters, parents and grandparents. Antiretroviral drugs could help some of the mine workers stay healthy longer, but the drugs have side effects of their own, they don't work for everyone, and they are certainly not a cure. Eventually, the family will need other kinds of help, including money for children's school fees and seeds, small loans, or help finding jobs and business advice, so that survivors can start small enterprises.

Because the economies of so many African countries are in such a bad state, many small enterprises fail, so families affected by AIDS also require some sort of financial safety net to tide them over while they try again. In addition, families affected by HIV need education about their legal and human rights, especially regarding property rights and HIV-related employment discrimination, which is widespread in developing countries. Since laws protecting the rights of people with HIV currently exist almost nowhere in Africa, mechanisms must be found to create and enforce them at local and national levels. Communities affected by HIV also need information about how people can protect themselves from the virus, and they will also need reliable supplies of condoms, which are still, twenty years into the AIDS epidemic, not easily and cheaply available everywhere.

Overemphasis on the medical aspects of AIDS in Africa probably arises from the tendency to see the problems of the developing world as reflections of problems in the West. But many small African AIDS groups see AIDS quite differently. They provide a wide range of social support and HIV prevention services, in addition to rudimentary care for AIDS patients. Most of these projects rely at present on dedicated volunteers and shoestring budgets, and there are not nearly enough of them to help everyone. Emphasizing access to AIDS drugs alone risks bypassing much of the very good work that these groups are already doing.

A strong case can be made that the pharmaceutical companies should either donate their drugs to Africa entirely for free or permit the use of generics, in exchange for some guarantee that their markets in industrialized countries will be protected. The companies can well afford to do this. A similarly strong case can be made that projects like the Faraja Trust in Morogoro, Tanzania, or the Friends of Street Children Project in Kampala, Uganda—to name just two of thousands of such groups in East Africa alone—should get most of the support from the Global Fund. Antiretrovirals could then be part of such programs whenever feasible.

The governing board of the Global Fund seems to recognize the importance of both national health systems and non-governmental programs that strive to meet the complex and specific needs of particular communities. Under the fund's guidelines made public at the end of January 2002, National AIDS Coordinating Councils, quasi-governmental bodies that include members from non-governmental organizations, will submit proposals to the fund, and the money will be disbursed to the government, usually the Ministry of Health, which will then pass the money on to non-governmental entities. However, there are already concerns that many groups will be over-looked. Cronyism and corruption, perennial problems with international aid in general, will also have to be addressed, but as yet, it is not clear how this will be done, or how the spending will be monitored.

Addressing the AIDS crisis in Africa will require an emphasis on more than antiretroviral drugs alone, important as they are. What sub-Saharan Africa seems to need even more than it needs AIDS drugs is the improvement of its health care systems, the creation of livelihoods for families impoverished by AIDS illnesses and deaths, and the alleviation of the loneliness, poverty, and despair that are likely to motivate risky sexual behavior. The Global Fund cannot deal with all this on its own. Until scientists discover an effective vaccine to prevent HIV infection, sustained relief from the African AIDS epidemic may depend on the subcontinent's social and economic stability, which in turn will depend on better governance by Africa's leaders. But it will also depend critically on greater support for Africa from the international community, which could begin by establishing fairer terms of trade for African farmers and debt relief programs that are not tied to the same harsh conditions—such as under-investment in African institutions, especially those devoted to health and education, and reduced government support for nascent African business enterprises that need to be nurtured—that have combined with local corruption and mismanagement to undermine African development.

Nevertheless, it is of enormous importance that the Global Fund succeed, not only because it could reduce much human suffering, but also because it could advance the credibility of new mechanisms to manage the negative consequences of globalization. If the fund's performance were to generate cynicism, it could undermine similar efforts in other areas. If successful, it could become a model for global governance in the future.

RICHARD STEARNS

President of World Vision

Women and Orphans: The Hidden Faces of AIDS

Adapted from a speech to supporters attending the World Vision Forum
New York City
May 18, 2002

Two thousand years after Jesus gave the church the parable of the Good Samaritan, we are still asking the question, "Who is my neighbor?" And we're still getting the answer wrong.

This simple-yet-most-profound parable speaks to the AIDS epidemic, a scourge that already has killed twenty million people, robbed thirteen million children of parents, and turned ten million wives into widows—many of them sick and desperate to find someone to care for their children when they die, too.

Jesus used this parable to challenge the religious establishment of his day. Today, the parable compels us to challenge our own community of faith, an American Church that largely is ignoring the AIDS pandemic. We must respond with our heads, with our hearts, and with our hands in practical compassion.

The story begins in Luke 10:25 when an "expert in the law" challenges Jesus—attempting to engage in a battle of the mind, to expose Jesus's theology as defective. Jesus turned the encounter into an examination of the heart.

The scholar asks a theological question: "Teacher, what shall I do to inherit eternal life?"[1]

Jesus responds in kind, "What is written in the law?"[2]

The lawyer's answer was a conventional reference to the Old Testament law from Leviticus and Deuteronomy, "'You shall love the Lord your God with all your heart, with all your soul, with all your strength, and with all your mind,' and 'your neighbor as yourself.'"[3]

Jesus replies, "You have answered rightly; do this and you will live."[4]

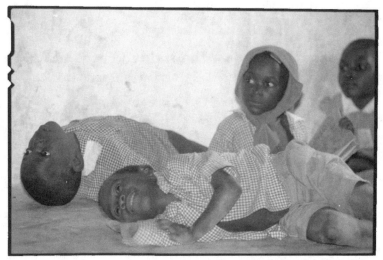

Courtesy of Jonathan W. Rodgers

Jesus brought the debate from the *thinking* to the *doing*. In other words, right thinking must be accompanied by right doing. The thought that he must change his behavior apparently troubled the man, so he asked a follow-up question: "And who is my neighbor?"[5]

This question is perhaps one of the most profound in all of Scripture. Even today, the answer defines truly Christian communities around the world.

Jesus' answer, in the form of the parable of the Good Samaritan, reverberates across the centuries as one of the most foundational and universal tenets of moral law, a lesson Jesus demonstrates through the actions of the four main characters: the victim, the priest, the Levite, and the Samaritan.

The Victim: The Man Who Was Beaten by Robbers

The one thing that is clear is that he was in dire need: beaten, wounded, bleeding—and possibly dying. We're not certain of his ethnicity or nationality. We don't know why he was beaten. He may have been an "innocent" victim, unjustly attacked. He may have been a robber, beaten by fellow thieves. Perhaps he was engaged in some illicit activity and was beaten as a result. Or perhaps he was just careless and had traveled irresponsibly alone at night along a dangerous road. The point is that we do not know. Jesus did not feel that it was relevant whether the man who had been beaten was at fault.

Here is raised one of the critical moral questions with regard to the victims of AIDS: Should we distinguish between those who became victims because of sinful behavior and those who were innocent victims? I believe that one of the reasons the Christian community has not taken a leading role in the fight against AIDS is this issue of judgment. We distinguish between the "innocent" victims, such as children infected or orphaned by their parents, and the "guilty," such as prostitutes and the promiscuous.

In truth, we are bound by Scripture to respond to all those "beaten" and "left by the side of the road" by this devastating virus.

Scripture makes clear who has the right and the responsibility to judge: It is God, not us. Yet we judge people with AIDS. We conveniently forget that we all would be dead if we faced such a certain death for any of our sins—including indifference to those who are suffering.

That sin, of course, is the only one Jesus condemns in the story of the Good Samaritan, and is embodied in the next two characters in the drama.

The Priest and the Levite: The Embodiment of Indifference

They represent the religious establishment of the day. Today, they might be a pastor and a seminary professor, practitioners of the faith and well-schooled in the law. We are told that they *saw* the man and yet they passed by on the other side of the road, unwilling to help. They knew what was right, but they failed to act.

Peter Singer, an ethicist at Princeton University, holds some of the most radical views of any modern-day philosopher—views that are morally shocking to a Christian audience. Yet his writing challenges us to think through the ethical implications of our behavior, particularly where inconsistencies exist between our beliefs and our actions, between knowing and doing.

He tells a parable very similar to that of the Good Samaritan: He uses the issue of poverty in his reasoning, but we could just as easily substitute the problem of AIDS.[6]

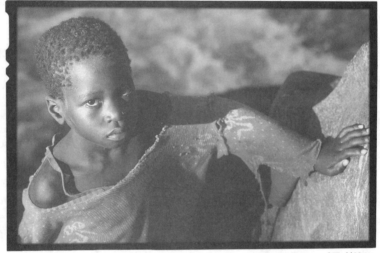

Courtesy of World Vision

The path from the library at my university to the humanities lecture theater passes a shallow ornamental pond. Suppose that on my way to give a lecture I notice that a small child has fallen in and is in danger of drowning. Would anyone deny that I ought to wade in and pull the child out?

This will mean getting my clothes muddy, and either canceling my lecture or delaying it until I can find something dry to change into; but compared with the avoidable death of a child this is insignificant.

A plausible principle that would support the judgment that I ought to pull the child out is this: if it is in our power to prevent something very bad from happening, without thereby sacrificing anything of comparable moral significance, we ought to do it. This principle seems uncontroversial.

Singer goes on to suggest that failing to save the child is the moral equivalent to killing the child. But few of us will see a child drowning in a pond, or a man beaten by the side of the road. He continues: *Nevertheless, [this principle] is deceptive. If it were seriously acted upon, our lives and our world would be fundamentally changed.*

For the principle applies, not just to rare situations in which one can save a child from a pond, but to the everyday situation in which we can assist those living in absolute poverty. Not to help would be wrong, whether or not it is intrinsically equivalent to killing.

Peter Singer wrestles with the question, "Who is my neighbor?" And, the logical follow-up question, "What is my responsibility toward him?" He is advocating the same radical thought as Jesus: Walking by on the other side of the road is wrong. This connection of belief to action seems simplistically obvious to us as Christians. Singer is not saying anything new. But, too often, beliefs fail to translate into action.

In 2001, World Vision commissioned a study through the Barna Research Group to determine the willingness of the Christian community to get involved in fighting the AIDS epidemic. When evangelical Christians were asked whether they would be willing to donate money to help children orphaned by AIDS, only 7 percent answered that they definitely would. More than half said that they probably or definitely would *not* help. Evangelicals were even less likely to support *education* efforts to help prevent AIDS.[7]

The survey found that by many measures, non-Christians were more inclined to help than those who claim to be followers of Jesus, in both spirit and word!

Here again is the gap between knowing and doing. My pastor, Gary Gulbranson[8], said one Sunday, "It's not what you believe that counts. It's what you believe enough to do." The priest and the Levite had the right beliefs, but they were unwilling to do what those beliefs logically dictated.

The book of James says it eloquently and succinctly: "But be doers of the word, and not hearers only, deceiving yourselves."[9] A chapter later, James is more explicit when he says:

> What does it profit, my brethren, if someone says he has faith but does not have works? Can faith save him? If a brother or sister is naked and destitute of daily food, and one of you says to them, "Depart in peace, be warmed and filled," but you do not give them the things which are needed for the body, what does it profit? Thus also faith by itself, if it does not have works, is dead.[10]

In light of this, how should the Christian community respond to the victims of HIV / AIDS? The fourth character of Jesus' parable shows us.

The Samaritan: The Hero of the Story

The Samaritans were despised by the Jews. They were considered heretical and unclean. Jews would not associate with them. Jesus's introduction of the Samaritan into this parable would have been shocking to the expert in the law, and the contrast between the compassion of the unclean Samaritan and the "righteous" priest and Levite scandalous.

We are told that this Samaritan saw the man at the side of the road "and took pity on him." He bandaged his wounds and poured oil and wine upon them as a salve. He put the man on his own donkey and transported him to an inn and left money for his care. And he promised to return to check up on the man again. It was not a minimal response. Rather, it was a complete engagement.

The Samaritan had compassion, which translated into action. Jesus turns the question back on the expert in the law, asking, "So which of these three do you think was neighbor to him who fell among the thieves?"[11]

The man could not even bring himself to say the word "Samaritan," and answers instead "He who showed mercy on him."[12]

The Samaritans of the AIDS crisis seem just as unlikely to today's religious establishment:

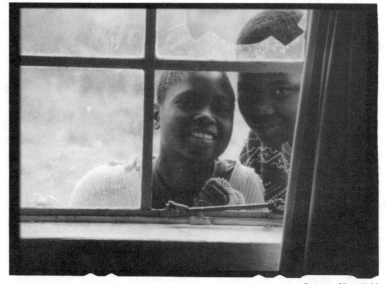

Courtesy of Pam Kidd

- The homosexual community
- Hollywood
- Political liberals
- The U.S. Government
- The United Nations
- Secular humanitarian organizations
- The Bill and Melinda Gates Foundation

And who would expect a rock star to be leading the charge? Bono, lead singer of the group U2, may be doing more to address the AIDS crisis than any other single person in the world. When addressing a group of Christians in Washington, Bono asked, "Will American Christians stand by as an entire continent dies for 'small money'?" A tough question.

The Lesson for the Church

Years from now, the AIDS pandemic will be judged as one of those rare crossroads in human history, where everything that comes after it will be seen through its lens. Every generation struggles with events and crises that ultimately define it. Every generation has its sins—of commission and omission. The lens of history can be brutally honest in its judgment.

How could American pioneers justify their treatment of Native Americans? How could pre-Civil-War America have tolerated slavery? How could churches in America have turned a blind eye to racial discrimination in the '40s and '50s? These are the kinds of questions that history asks, and the questions that children and grandchildren ask of their parents and grandparents. "Why didn't you act?" "How could you remain silent?"

No one can predict the outcome of the AIDS crisis with certainty—whether vaccines will be found or whether the epidemic will be somehow stopped ten, fifty or one hundred years from today. No one can predict how many men, women and children will die, or how many orphans and widows will suffer in obscurity. No one can predict how this generation will be viewed through that lens of history. But I know that we cannot remain silent, and I am certain of what Jesus would have us do.

A call to action. I am certain about God's expectations of His people. I am certain that God sees these widows and orphans as our neighbors, lying beaten and bleeding on the side of the road, helpless and needing our help. And I am certain that He calls us to stop, show compassion, comfort them, bind up their wounds and see that they and their children are cared for.

In Matthew 25 we hear described the spectacular scene at the last judgment when all of the nations will be gathered before the master and we hear these remarkable words:

'Come, you blessed of My Father, inherit the kingdom prepared for you from the foundation of the world: for I was hungry and you gave Me food; I was thirsty and you gave Me drink; I was a stranger and you took Me in; I was

naked and you clothed Me; I was sick and you visited Me; I was in prison
and you came to Me.' Then the righteous will answer Him, saying, 'Lord,
when did we see You hungry and feed You, or thirsty and give You drink?
When did we see You a stranger and take You in, or naked and clothe You?
Or when did we see You sick, or in prison, and come to You?' And the King
will answer and say to them, 'Assuredly, I say to you, inasmuch as you did
it to one of the least of these My brethren, you did it to Me.' [15]

Mother Teresa saw Christ in every dying beggar or leper she
served. She once said this of these broken and forgotten souls: "I see
the face of Jesus in disguise—sometimes a most distressing disguise."
She understood that in serving the "least of these," she was not serving the loathsome and despicable, but was privileged to serve the
person of Jesus Himself.

Henri Nouwen, the priest, professor, and philosopher pointed
out that "God rejoices. Not because the problems of the world have
been solved, not because all human pain and suffering have come to
an end, nor because thousands of people have been converted and
are now praising Him for His goodness. No, God rejoices because
one of His children who was lost has been found."[14]

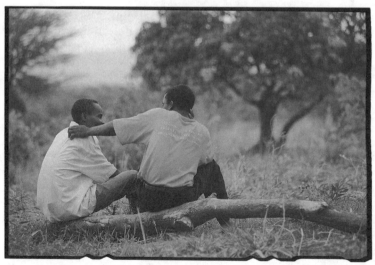

Courtesy of World Vision

We can reach out to the one: the one widow, the one orphan, the one father, the one mother. We can demonstrate the love of Christ to these dear children who have lost their parents. We can encourage right behaviors so they can avoid their parents' fate. We can come alongside grandparents, aunts and uncles trying to raise these orphaned children. And we can comfort the sick and dying and offer them hope for a new life in Christ. We can reach out to the "least of these."

How? By advocating for right theology in our churches and right policies by our government. By praying for people with AIDS, for the children they leave behind, and for their caregivers. By volunteering with local organizations serving people affected by HIV/AIDS. And by supporting our brothers and sisters in Africa and elsewhere in their efforts to stop this epidemic and care for those whose lives already have been shattered.

Jesus ends the parable of the Good Samaritan with a powerful challenge. When he asked the expert in the law which of the three men had been a neighbor to the man who fell into the hands of robbers, he answers with a new understanding: "The one who had mercy on him."

Jesus then looks at this man and concludes what is perhaps the most powerful moral teaching in all of history with a command of just four words. Four words that reverberate through history. Four words that declare Christ's expectations of every Christian. Four words with the power to change the world.

"Go and do likewise."[15]

Written for The aWAKE Project.
Copyright © 2002 by Richard Stearns.

MARK SCHOOFS

Journalist, Pulitzer Prize Winner 2000

AIDS: The Agony of Africa
Part One: The Virus Creates a Generation of Orphans

They didn't call Arthur Chinaka out of the classroom. The principal and Arthur's uncle Simon waited until the day's exams were done before breaking the news: Arthur's father, his body wracked with pneumonia, had finally died of AIDS. They were worried that Arthur would panic, but at 17 years old, he didn't. He still had two days of tests, so while his father lay in the morgue, Arthur finished his exams. That happened in 1990. Then in 1992, Arthur's uncle Edward died of AIDS. In 1994, his uncle Richard died of AIDS. In 1996, his uncle Alex died of AIDS. All of them are buried on the homestead where they grew up and where their parents and Arthur still live, a collection of thatch-roofed huts in the mountains near Mutare, by Zimbabwe's border with Mozambique. But HIV hasn't finished with this family. In April, a fourth uncle lay coughing in his hut, and the virus had blinded Arthur's aunt Eunice, leaving her so thin and weak she couldn't walk without help. By September both were dead.

The most horrifying part of this story is that it is not unique. In Uganda, a business executive named Tonny, who asked that his last name not be used, lost two brothers and a sister to AIDS, while his wife lost her brother to the virus. In the rural hills of South Africa's KwaZulu Natal province, Bonisile Ngema lost her

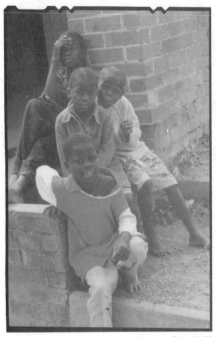

Courtesy of Pam Kidd

son and daughter-in-law, so she tries to support her granddaughter and her own aged mother by selling potatoes. Her dead son was the breadwinner for the whole extended family, and now *she* feels like an orphan.

In the morgue of Zimbabwe's Parirenyatwa Hospital, head mortician Paul Tabvemhiri opens the door to the large cold room that holds cadavers. But it's impossible to walk in because so many bodies lie on the floor, wrapped in blankets from their deathbeds or dressed in the clothes they died in.

Along the walls, corpses are packed two to a shelf. In a second cold-storage area, the shelves are narrower, so Tabvemhiri faces a grisly choice: He can stack the bodies on top of one another, which squishes the face and makes it hard for relatives to identify the body, or he can leave the cadavers out in the hall, unrefrigerated. He refuses to deform bodies, and so a pair of corpses lie outside on gurneys behind a curtain. The odor of decomposition is faint but clear.

Have they always had to leave bodies in the hall? "No, no, no," says Tabvemhiri, who has worked in the morgue since 1976. "Only in the last five or six years," which is when AIDS deaths here took off. Morgue records show that the number of cadavers has almost tripled since the start of Zimbabwe's epidemic, and there's been a change in *who* is dying: "The young ones," says Tabvemhiri, "are coming in bulk."

The wide crescent of East and Southern Africa that sweeps down from Mount Kenya and around the Cape of Good Hope is the hardest-hit AIDS region in the world. Here, the virus is cutting down more and more of Africa's most energetic and productive people, adults aged 15 to 49. The slave trade also targeted people in their prime, killing or sending into bondage perhaps 25 million people. But that happened over four centuries. Only 17 years have passed since AIDS was first found in Africa, on the shores of Lake Victoria, yet according to the Joint United Nations Programme on HIV/AIDS (UNAIDS), the virus has already killed more than 11 million sub-Saharan Africans. More than 22 million others are infected.

Only 10 percent of the world's population lives south of the Sahara, but the region is home to two-thirds of the world's HIV-positive people, and it has suffered more than 80 percent of all AIDS deaths.

Last year, the combined wars in Africa killed 200,000 people. AIDS killed 10 times that number. Indeed, more people succumbed to HIV last year than to any other cause of death on this continent, including malaria. And the carnage has only begun.

Unlike ebola or influenza, AIDS is a slow plague, gestating in individuals for five to 10 years before killing them. Across East and Southern Africa, more than 13 percent of adults are infected with HIV, according to UNAIDS. And in three countries, including Zimbabwe, more than a quarter of adults carry the virus. In some districts, the rates are even higher: In one study, a staggering 59 percent of women attending prenatal clinics in rural Beitbridge, Zimbabwe, tested HIV-positive.

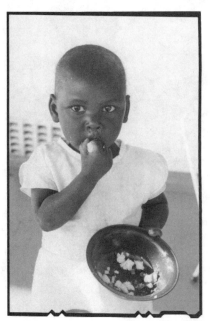

Courtesy of Pam Kidd

Life expectancy in more than a dozen African countries

"will soon be 17 years shorter because of AIDS—47 years instead of 64," says Callisto Madavo, the World Bank's vice president for Africa. HIV "is quite literally robbing Africa of a quarter of our lives."

In the West, meanwhile, the HIV death rate has dropped steeply thanks to powerful drug cocktails that keep the disease from progressing. These regimens must be taken for years, probably for life, and they can cost more than $10,000 per patient per year. Yet in many of the hardest-hit African countries, the total per capita health-care budget is less than $10.

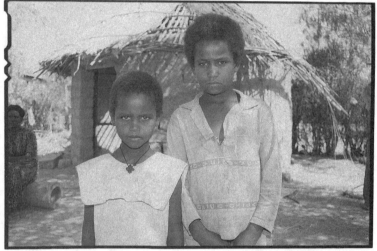

Courtesy of World Vision

Many people—in Africa as well as the West—shrug off this stark disparity, contending that it is also true for other diseases. But it isn't. Drugs for the world's major infectious killers—tuberculosis, malaria, and diarrheal diseases—have been subsidized by the international community for years, as have vaccines for childhood illnesses such as polio and measles. But even at discounted prices, the annual cost of putting every African with HIV on triple combination therapy would exceed $150 billion, so the world is letting a leading infectious killer for which treatment exists mow down millions.

That might be more palatable if there were a Marshall Plan for AIDS prevention to slow the virus's spread. But a recent study by UNAIDS and Harvard shows that in 1997 international donor countries devoted $150 million to AIDS prevention in Africa. That's less than the cost of the movie *Wild Wild West*.

Meanwhile, the epidemic is seeping into Central and West Africa. More than a tenth of adults in Côte d'Ivoire are infected. Frightening increases have been documented in Yaoundé and Douala, the largest cities in Cameroon. And in Nigeria—the continent's most populous country—past military dictatorships let the AIDS control program wither, even while the prevalence of HIV has climbed to almost one in every 20 adults.

Quite simply, AIDS is on track to dwarf every catastrophe in Africa's recorded history. It is stunting development, threatening the economy, and transforming cultural traditions.

Epidemics are never merely biological. Even as HIV changes African society, it spreads by exploiting current cultural and economic conditions. "The epidemic gets real only in a context," says Elhadj Sy, head of UNAIDS's East and Southern Africa Team. "In Africa, people wake up in the morning and try to survive—but the way they do that often puts them at risk for infection." For example, men migrate to cities in search of jobs; away from their wives and families for months on end, they seek sexual release with women who, bereft of property and job skills, are selling their bodies to feed themselves and their children. Back home, wives who ask their husbands to wear condoms risk being accused of sleeping around; in African cultures, it's usually the man who dictates when and how sex happens.

Challenging such cultural and economic forces requires political will, but most African governments have been shockingly derelict. Lacking leadership, ordinary Africans have been slow to confront the disease. Few companies, for example, have comprehensive AIDS programs. And many families still refuse to acknowledge that HIV is killing their relatives, preferring to say that the person died of TB or some other opportunistic illness. Doctors often collude in this denial. "Just the other day," says a high-ranking Zimbabwean physician who spoke on condition of anonymity, "I wrote AIDS on a death certificate and then crossed it out. I thought, 'I'll just be stigmatizing this person, because no one else puts AIDS as the cause of death, even when that's what it is.'"

Why is AIDS worse in sub-Saharan Africa than anywhere else in the world? Partly because of denial; partly because the virus almost certainly originated here, giving it more time to spread; but largely because Africa was weakened by 500 years of slavery and colonialism. Indeed, historians lay much of the blame on colonialism for Africa's many corrupt and autocratic governments, which hoard resources that could fight the epidemic. Africa, conquered and denigrated, was never allowed to incorporate international innovations on its own terms, as, for example, Japan did.

This colonial legacy poisons more than politics. Some observers attribute the spread of HIV to polygamy, a tradition in many African cultures. But job migration, urbanization, and social dislocation have created a caricature of traditional polygamy. Men have many partners not through marriage but through prostitution or sugar-daddy arrangements that lack the social glue of the old polygamy.

Of course, the worst legacy of whites in Africa is poverty, which fuels the epidemic in countless ways. Having a sexually transmitted disease multiplies the chances of spreading and contracting HIV, but few Africans obtain effective treatment because the clinic is too expensive or too far away. Africa's wealth was either funneled to the West or restricted to white settlers who barred blacks from full participation in the economy. In apartheid South Africa, blacks were either not educated at all or taught only enough to be servants. Now, as the country suffers one of the world's most explosive AIDS epidemics, illiteracy hampers prevention. Indeed, AIDS itself is rendering Africa still more vulnerable to any future catastrophe, continuing history's vicious cycle.

Yet AIDS is not merely a tale of despair. Increasingly, Africans are banding together—usually with meager resources—to care for their sick, raise their orphans, and prevent the virus from claiming more of their loved ones. Their efforts offer hope. For while a crisis of this magnitude can disintegrate society, it can also unify it. "To solve HIV," says Sy, "you must involve yourself: your attitudes and behavior and beliefs. It touches upon the most fundamental social and cultural things-procreation and death."

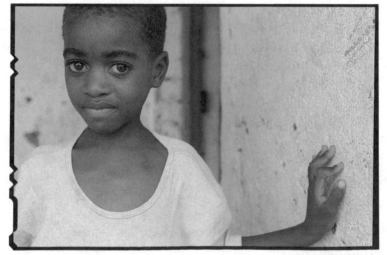

Courtesy of World Vision

AIDS is driving a new candor about sex—as well as new efforts to control it, through virginity testing and campaigns that advocate sticking to one partner. And slowly, fitfully, it is also giving women more power. The death toll is scaring women into saying no to sex or insisting on condoms. And as widows proliferate, people are beginning to see the harm in denying them the right to inherit property.

The epidemic is also transforming kinship networks, which have been the heart of most African cultures. Orphans, for example, have always been enfolded into the extended family. But more than 7 million children in sub-Saharan Africa have lost one or both parents, and the virus is also killing their aunts and uncles, depriving them of foster parents and leaving them to live with often feeble grandparents. In response, communities across Africa are volunteering to help orphans through home visits and, incredibly, by sharing the very little they have. Such volunteerism is both a reclaiming of communal traditions and their adaptation into new forms of civil society.

But even heroic efforts can't stop the damage that's already occurred here in the hills where Arthur Chinaka lost his father and uncles. The worst consequence of this epidemic is not the dead, but the living they leave behind.

Rusina Kasongo lives a couple of hills over from Chinaka. Like a lot of elderly rural folk who never went to school, Kasongo can't calculate how old she is, but she can count her losses: Two of her sons, one of her daughters, and all their spouses died of AIDS, and her husband died in an accident. Alone, she is rearing 10 orphaned children.

"Sometimes the children go out and come home very late," says Kasongo, "and I'm afraid they'll end up doing the same thing as Tanyaradzwa." That's the daughter who died of AIDS; she had married twice, the first time in a shotgun wedding. Now, the eldest orphan, 17-year-old Fortunate, already has a child but not a husband.

Few people have conducted more research on AIDS orphans than pediatrician Geoff Foster, who founded the Family AIDS Caring Trust (FACT). It was Foster who documented that more than half of Zimbabwe's orphans are being cared for by grandparents, usually grandmothers who had nursed their own children to the grave. But even this fragile safety net won't be there for many of the next generation of orphans.

"Perhaps one-third of children in Zimbabwe will have lost a father or mother—or both—to AIDS," says Foster. They are more likely to be poor, he explains, more likely to be deprived of education, more likely to be abused or neglected or stigmatized, more likely to be seething with all the needs that make it more likely that a person will have unsafe sex. "But when they get HIV and die, who cares for their children? Nobody, because they're orphans, so by definition their kids have no grandparents. It's just like the virus itself. In the body, HIV gets into the defense system and knocks it out. It does that sociologically, too. It gets into the extended family support system and decimates it."

Foster's chilling realization is dawning on other people who work in fields far removed from HIV. This year, South African crime researcher Martin Schönteich published a paper that begins by noting, "In a decade's time every fourth South African will be aged between 15 and 24. It is at this age group where people's propensity to commit crime is at its highest. At about the same time there will be a boom in South Africa's orphan population as the AIDS epidemic takes its toll." While some causes of crime can be curtailed, Schönteich writes, "Other causes, such as large numbers of juveniles in the general population, and a high proportion of children brought up without adequate parental supervision, are beyond the control of the state." His conclusion: "No amount of state spending on the criminal justice system will be able to counter this harsh reality."

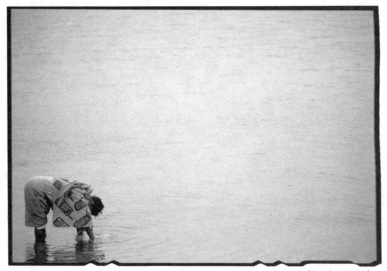

Courtesy of Jonathan W. Rodgers

More AIDS and more crime are among the most dramatic consequences of the orphan explosion. But Nengomasha Willard sees damage that is harder to measure. Willard teaches 11- and 12-year-olds at Saint George's Primary School, located near the Chinakas and the Kasongos. Fifteen of Willard's 42 pupils have lost one or both of their parents, but he's particularly worried about one of his students who lost his father and then, at his mother's funeral, cried inconsolably. "He doesn't want to participate," says Willard. "He just wants to be alone."

"I see thousands of children sitting in a corner," says Foster. "The impact is internalized—it's depression, being withdrawn." In Africa, says Foster, the focus on poverty eclipses research into psychological issues, but he has published disturbing evidence of abuse—emotional, physical, and sexual. Meanwhile, the orphan ranks keep swelling. "We're talking 10 percent who will have lost both parents, maybe 15 percent. Twenty-five percent who will have lost a mother. What does that do to a society, especially an impoverished society?"

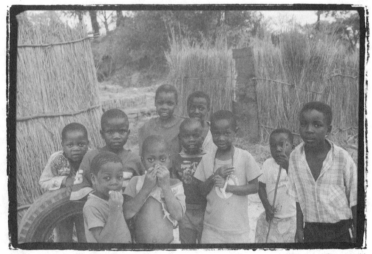

Courtesy of Pam Kidd

Among his students, Willard has noticed that some of the orphans come to school without shoes or, in Zimbabwe's cold winter, without a sweater. Sometimes their stepfamilies put them last on the list, but often it's because grandmothers can't scrape together enough money.

Among economists, there has been a quiet debate over whether HIV will harm the economy. Some think it won't. With unemployment rates in sub-Saharan Africa between 30 and 70 percent, they reason that there are plenty of people to replenish labor losses. One scenario is that economic growth might slacken, but population growth will also dwindle, so per capita GNP might hold steady or even rise. Then, says Helen Jackson, executive director of the Southern Africa AIDS Information Dissemination Service (SAfAIDS), Africa might face the grotesque irony of "an improvement in some macroeconomic indicators, but the exact opposite at the level of households and human suffering."

But evidence is mounting that the economy will suffer. Between 20 and 30 percent of workers in South Africa's gold mining industry—the mainstay of that country's economy—are estimated to be HIV-positive, and replacing these workers will cut into the industry's productivity. In Kenya, a new government report predicts that per capita income could sink by 10 percent over the next five years. In Côte d'Ivoire, a teacher dies every school day.

Then there are the effects that can't be quantified. "What does AIDS do for the image of Africa?" asks Tony Barnett, a veteran researcher on the economic impact of AIDS. To lure investors, the continent already has to battle underdevelopment and racism, but now, he says, many people will see Africa as "diseased, sexually diseased. It chimes in with so many stereotypes."

Beneath the corporate economy, millions of Africans subsist by cultivating their own small plot of land. When someone in the family comes down with AIDS, the other members have to spend time caring for that person, which means less time cultivating crops. And when death comes, the family loses a crucial worker. Studies have documented that among rural AIDS-stricken families, food production falls, savings dwindle, and children are more likely to be undernourished.

For Kasongo and her 10 orphans, food is a constant problem, but now it has become even harder. On her way back from the fields, carrying a basket of maize on her head, Kasongo tripped and fell. Her knee is swollen, her back is aching, and cultivating the fields is close to impossible. Here, under the radar of macroeconomic indicators, Kasongo's ordeal shows how AIDS is devastating Africa.

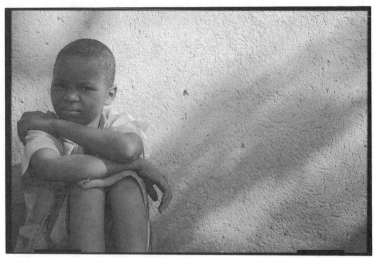

Courtesy of World Vision

This is the context in which one of Africa's most agonizing debates is taking place: Should doctors administer drugs to pregnant women that sharply reduce the chances that a baby will be born with HIV? So far, the debate has centered on the cost of the drugs, but a new, inexpensive regimen has pushed thornier arguments to the surface.

The "vaccine for babies," as it is sometimes called, does not treat the mother and so does nothing to reduce the chances the baby will become an orphan. That's why Uganda's Major Rubaramira Ruranga, a well-known activist who is himself infected with HIV, opposes it. "Many children in our countries die of malnutrition, even with both parents," he argues. "Without parents, it's almost certain they'll die."

Isn't it impossible to know the fate of any given child and presumptuous to decide it in advance? "That's sentimental," he snaps. Even Foster, who believes "every child has a right to be born without HIV," wonders whether the money is best spent on the "technical fix" of giving drugs to the pregnant women. The medicine is only a part of the cost, for women can infect their children during breast feeding, which raises expensive problems such as providing formula and teaching mothers how to use it safely in places where clean water may not exist. Would all that money, Foster wonders, be better spent alleviating the root causes of why women get infected in the first place? "It's very difficult to stand up and make such an argument because you get portrayed as a beast," he says. In fact, such arguments testify to how the epidemic is forcing Africans to grapple with impossible choices.

Weston Tizora is one of thousands of Africans who are trying to give orphans a decent life. Just 25 years old, Tizora started as a gardener at Saint Augustine's Mission and threw himself into volunteering in the mission's AIDS program, called Kubatana, a Shona word meaning "together." Next year he will take over the program's leadership from its founder, British nurse Sarah Hinton. Kubatana's 37 volunteers care for homebound patients, and they help raise orphans by, for example, bringing food to Rusina Kasongo's brood.

Just a few steps from Kasongo live Cloud and Joseph Tineti. They're 14 and 11, respectively, and the oldest person in their home is their 15-year-old brother. They are, in the language of AIDS workers, a child-headed household. Who's in charge? "No one," Joseph answers—and it shows. Their one-room shack is strewn with dirty clothes, unwashed dishes, broken chairs. On the table, a roiling mass of ants feasts on pumpkin seeds and some kind of dried leaves.

The troubles run deeper. Their father, who had divorced their mother before she died, lives in nearby Mutare. Does he bring food? "Yes," says Joseph, "every week." It's not true, Tizora maintains. Kubatana members have even talked with the police in their effort to convince the father to take in his children or at least support them. But the police did not act, explains Tizora, because the father is unemployed and struggling to provide for the family of his second wife. Once a month—sometimes not even that often— he brings small amounts of food, so the orphans depend on donations from Kubatana volunteers.

But if little Joseph's version isn't true, it's what an orphaned kid would want: a father who at least brings food, stops by frequently, and acts a little like a dad. And his mother: What does Joseph remember of her? The question is too much, and he starts crying.

Kubatana volunteers are supposed to look after the Tineti orphans, so why is their home so unkempt? There used to be two volunteers in this area, explains Tizora. One has been reassigned to work in the nearby mining village, ravaged by AIDS. The other has been away at her parents' home for two months, attending to a family funeral and to her own late-stage pregnancy.

And everyone in these villages has their hands full. Standing in a valley, Tizora points to the hillsides around him and says, "There are orphans in that home, and the one over there, and there by the gum trees. And see where there's that white house? They're taking care of orphans there, too." By the time he finishes, he has pointed out about half of the homesteads. When the Kubatana program started, in 1992, volunteers identified 20 orphans. Now they have registered 3,000. In many parts of Africa, notes Jackson of SAfAIDS, "It has actually become the norm to have orphaned children in the household rather than the exception."

Foster makes some quick calculations: Given the number of volunteers in the Kubatana program, there's no way they can care for all their orphans. So when a volunteer gets pregnant, has a family emergency, or gets sick, kids like Cloud and Joseph fall through the cracks. Says Foster: "You can't lose a quarter of your adult population in 10 years without catastrophic consequences."

In his office, Tizora has a wall of photographs showing the original 20 orphans. One is a girl who looks about 12. She lost her parents and then she lost the grandma who was caring for her. At that point, she started refusing to go to school, hiding on the way there. Now, she's run away and, Tizora says, "we don't know where she is."

RECAH THEODOSIOU

Journalist

The Friendly City

From the airplane window, through the glare of the sun, it could be any coastal city. Downtown nestles behind the harbor. Hotels and beachfront apartments to the left reflect the bright sands; and industry occupies the coastline to the right. Suburbs, arranged neatly along asphalt grids, stretch out behind. The city of Port Elizabeth encircles a bay on the southeast coast of Africa. The glistening Indian Ocean calmly laps at her shores.

From the car window, on the drive from the airport, Africa becomes subtly evident in the details. An aged man herds cattle between suburban homes; at busy intersections, barefoot children beg drivers for money; traffic is brought to a crawl behind a donkey cart; and main thoroughfares are lined with men holding up the tools of their trade in hope.

These details hint at what wasn't noticed from above. Multi-colored specks scattered across open land in and on the city outskirts. Not all homes are on the grid. From the asphalt the crude shelters, which hundreds of thousands of adults, children, and babies call home, dot the veld as far as can be seen. Discarded corrugated iron, cardboard, plastic, wood, are the roofs and walls. No electricity, no water.

From the glassless window of a shack, the world is inhospitable. There is no money for basics like warm clothing, warm bedding,

161

and enough food. And as if crippling poverty is not enough to have to cope with, HIV—the virus that causes AIDS—is creeping through almost every shantytown door. Most of those infected in these living conditions suffer and slowly die of the incurable disease at home without any pain-relieving drugs.

In a city of over one million people, the sole care provider for AIDS victims is the House of Resurrection Haven, which can only afford to admit nine adults and twelve children at one time. The four cash-strapped government hospitals in the Port Elizabeth area are most often forced to turn adults, children, and even babies with AIDS away to make space and resources available to those with curable ailments.

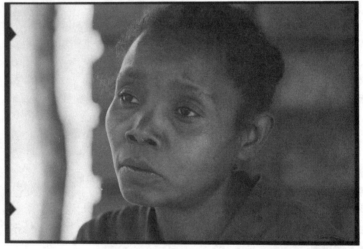

Courtesy of World Vision

"We have a limited budget, so when a baby gets bad, like with pneumonia, we won't admit it for the second time—we tell the mother to take it home and let it die," a pediatrics head at one of the hospitals told the city's *East Cape Weekend* newspaper. He explains: "We can only treat the secondary infection, but that's like treating hypertension with a headache tablet."

House of Resurrection Haven head, registered nurse Maggie

Williams, says as far as she knows the only other free AIDS care in the city is that received by the 213 people cared for in their homes by the privately-funded St. Francis Hospice. Over 400,000 of the city's population is unemployed, and people working in the impoverished communities estimate that at least one in every four is HIV-positive.

At night cold seeps through the bare earth floor; during the day the sun bakes the corrugated iron roof. Lying on blankets on the floor, a mattress if lucky, an old bed if luckier, those with AIDS fight a losing battle against infections. Viruses carried by the many family and friends sleeping in the shack at night, starvation, and extreme temperature changes make the immune system ineffective.

Death is usually painfully slow. It can take two to three weeks for the weakest body infected with the strongest HIV, according to Mrs. Williams. Most grow thinner and thinner, and more and more fatigued, as tuberculosis or pneumonia, skin cancer, meningitis, thrush, herpes, and bacterial infections attack the body. "Most die coughing uncontrollably and with chronic diarrhea no amount of hydration can help," she says.

Drugs can ease the inhumane pain and suffering of AIDS, and, combined with a healthy diet, can considerably prolong life. "Most people admitted to our haven are on their death-bed, and we manage to get 50 percent up and walking again." Mrs. Williams says she was recently convinced a woman infected by her husband, the only man she had ever had sexual relations with, was too far-gone for treatment to make any difference. "She couldn't even swallow food. I was convinced she wouldn't make it, but after a couple of weeks she left with a life expectancy of six months. She was very grateful to have that extra time with her children."

The only drugs available designed specifically to treat AIDS and prevent the spread of HIV, including mother-to-child transmission, are too expensive even for the haven. "The anti-retroviral drugs available in South Africa cost R3,000 (approximately $300 U.S.) for one month's treatment," says Mrs. Williams.

Yes, AIDS in Africa is predominantly transmitted through

heterosexual relations, but before the thought: "It's their own fault, they deserve the consequences" comes to mind, note that many of those infected are innocent. Many woman and children are infected through sexual assault, and babies contract AIDS in their HIV-infected mothers' wombs—born to die. Many other cases of HIV-infection occur due to ignorance about AIDS and how to prevent its transmission.

More than 50 percent of the House of Resurrection Haven's patients were infected through sexual assault. The stigma of rape results in many cases not being reported to police. Nevertheless, in 2001, there were 1,601 cases in the Port Elizabeth area. The common result: AIDS babies. A pediatrics head at one of the city's government hospitals told the local *East Cape Weekend* newspaper that at least two babies were diagnosed with AIDS every day at the hospital.

Other than government efforts and small private initiatives, the only AIDS education program in the impoverished communities of the Port Elizabeth area is Mpilo-Lwazi (translated Health-Knowledge), which reaches thousands of adults and over twenty thousand of their children. It falls under the Ubuntu Education Fund, a U.S.-based non-profit organization assisting twenty-two schools in these areas.

Ubuntu Education Fund founder and president, twenty-four-year-old Jacob Lief of Pennsylvania, says he feels Mpilo-Lwazi is a "drop in the ocean." He says, from his office in New Jersey: "It's disgraceful what we are doing as Americans. It's a joke. We're going to look back at the AIDS crisis in Africa and say: 'How didn't we do anything?' Americans think that because Africa is thousands of miles away, it's not our problem and that it's not going to affect us, but it will eventually catch up with us."

Mr. Lief says what scares him most about his work in Port Elizabeth is that death is a daily occurrence. "People are becoming numb to it. Entire weekends in the townships are spent attending funerals of friends and family. I quickly learned not to even try to make appointments with people on weekends." Mr. Lief says he recently heard that three members of a Port Elizabeth friend's family—his brother, sister-in-law, and eighteen-year-old niece—died of AIDS within five weeks. "The cemeteries are invading the townships. They are running out of space to bury their dead."

Despite the haven's selfless work, Mrs. Williams says she doesn't feel it's making any difference to the AIDS crisis in the city. "To stop myself from hitting my head against a wall, I have to remember that even if we help one person it's something. The twenty people at the haven are twenty less going without care. We desperately need to extend the haven and increase the number of staff. We can only afford four staff per twelve-hour shift. We're begging for funds everywhere and anywhere. The government only covers 10 percent of our annual R1-million (approximately $100,000 U.S.) turnover. The scary thing is this epidemic is just starting. When it really hits, people are going to get the shock of their lives. They think a couple of donations will absolve their conscience."

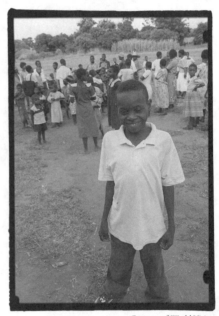

Courtesy of World Vision

According to official statistics there were only 5,004 HIV cases in Port Elizabeth in 2001. Mr. Lief says these statistics do not reflect the severity of the AIDS epidemic in the city. Most people with HIV and even AIDS don't know they have it, don't have access to HIV testing, and many don't *want* to know whether they have it or not. The social stigma attached to the disease makes the situation even worse. People don't want to tell anyone they are infected in fear of being ostracized by the terrified community, and even family, around them.

From the sidewalk, through the lens of a camera, the historic buildings downtown could be in any city. Port Elizabeth was founded by four thousand British settlers, who came by sea to the bay in 1820. These settlers became the first permanent British residents in South Africa. The city was named after the wife of the acting governor of the Cape Colony at the time.

From the game-viewing vehicle, the majestic Big Five—elephant, black rhino, buffalo, lion, and leopard—are a disturbing paradox to the pitiful circumstances of many of their human neighbors.

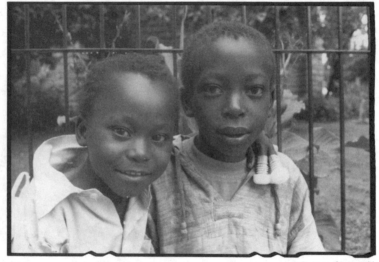

Courtesy of Pam Kidd

Yet, like the wildlife, the city's shack dwellers are vulnerable to the elements. Fortunately, nature in Port Elizabeth is fairly sympathetic. The climate is moderate all year round. The average temperature is 63 degrees Fahrenheit in summer and 77 degrees in winter. There are fewer rainy days and more sunshine hours than any coastal city in the country, and it is malaria-free.

This is small relief for the 43,000 people living in Kleinskool Squatter Camp, situated in the northern areas of Port Elizabeth. Eighty percent of the residents have no running water or proper sanitation.

Medical help is almost non-existent. The nearest government hospital is six miles away, and people wait for days before being attended to. One mobile clinic, only available to mothers with babies, visits the camp for two hours on Thursday and Friday mornings.

Reverend Boet Walker, who has run "Jesus is Lord Ministries" in Kleinskool for twelve years with his wife, Annatjie, says he has heard stories of people dying in the hospital's waiting room. Mrs. Williams says she heard of a woman with AIDS who was taken out of a hospital ward and left in a cold corridor overnight because there was not enough space for her. She died. "She might have been near the end, but a cold hospital corridor is no place for a sick person."

From a child's bright eyes, growing up in Kleinskool is a cruel survival game. Playing in the river situated alongside the camp often results in disease. The Chatty River serves as the community's garbage and sewer disposal. Home isn't even safe. "Three to four families can live in a three-room shack. This is an unhealthy situation because adults and children sleep together, and the result is often incest," says Rev. Walker. And there's never enough food. He says 25 percent of the children have sores on their bodies caused by malnutrition.

Despite the hopelessness, the broad white smiles and shiny creased eyes on the dark faces of children dressed in rags, kicking a punctured ball in the red sand outside a shack, bring brief warmth to the hearts of their mothers carrying buckets of water home—the children's baby sisters and brothers wrapped to their backs.

The unemployment rate in Kleinskool is 80 percent. The result is rampant crime, rape, and drugs in the area. "Many go to illegal bars when they have a bit of money to get drunk and forget about their problems," says Rev. Walker.

Harvest Christian Church in Port Elizabeth, which "Jesus is Lord Ministries" falls under, is trying to gather funds to set up an HIV/AIDS program in Kleinskool to help the community effectively deal with the disease. Harvest Christian Church resident social worker, twenty-four-year-old Becky Douglas-Jones, who is heading up the program, says it will offer counseling, education, and training to the community to care for family members with AIDS.

The innocent and ignorant in Port Elizabeth desperately need the world's help. The city does not have the funds needed to care for those dying of AIDS in inhumane pain, or to educate those fortunate enough not to be infected . . . yet.

Mrs. Williams says what the struggling House of Resurrection Haven needs most is prayer and that what people need to realize is that just $10 can help tremendously. "A very small amount can go a long way. To care for one person for a month costs us $300. That includes medicine, electricity, maintenance—everything.

She says the patients don't pay a cent for the care. Some of them don't even have clothing when they're admitted. "The other day a homeless man with AIDS, who was found almost dead under a bridge, was brought to us."

Jesus is Lord Ministries aims to compliment Harvest Christian Church's HIV/AIDS program by setting up a medical clinic, a soup kitchen and bakery, training workshop classrooms, and accommodation for visiting mission teams.

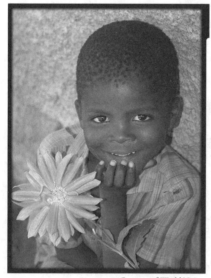
Courtesy of World Vision

"This whole project will cost R1,800,000 (approximately $180,000 U.S.). The plans are drawn, the land is bought, and the community has been trained to make the building blocks, which will be used for the new buildings," says Rev. Walker.

According to statistics, the average age of AIDS deaths is twenty-nine. Men and women beginning their own families and looking forward to watching their children grow up are faced with the heartache and guilt of leaving them with little hope in life. With one generation dying and the next left crippled, parenthood is cut short and childhood stunted.

Port Elizabeth, also known as the "Friendly City," is the fifth largest in South Africa in terms of population and the second largest in terms of area. It is a microcosm of urban life in South Africa. However, the situation in the vast rural areas of the country is worse. The little help to be found in cities is often non-existent beyond.

The HIV/AIDS epidemic in South Africa is a raging wildfire out of control. Over 4.7 million people are infected with AIDS and this number is expected to reach six million by 2010. By 2000 there was an approximate average of 300,000 AIDS-related deaths per year. There are an estimated 420,000 orphans, and by 2005 it is estimated there will be between 800,000 and one million orphans under the age of fifteen.

From outside Africa it's difficult to see the trees for the forest. The raging fire looks too widespread to quench. The key is to look beyond the forest to the individual trees. If one person at a time is educated or cared for, an entire continent can be saved.

Walking the streets of Africa's cities, brushing shoulders and coming eye-to-eye with its suffering makes the heart ache, but there isn't time to shed a tear. What right do the fortunate have to cry? Leave the crying for those starving and dying in Africa.

Written for The aWAKE Project.
Copyright © 2002 by Recah Theodosiou.

GREGORY BARZ

Ethnomusicologist

No One Will Listen to Us Unless We Bring Our Drums!: AIDS and Women's Music Performance in Uganda

Prelude

During a visit several years ago to the village of Kibaale-Busiki in eastern Uganda, I noticed a woman approach the farm of Centurio Balikoowa, my Ugandan research colleague, where I was conducting field research. The woman carried a small *akadongo* (a musical instrument often referred to as a "thumb piano") slung across her shoulder as she made her way toward us from the pathway through a banana field that led from a neighboring village. Several hours later as I concluded a recording session with the male village musicians, I noticed that the woman with the *akadongo* had joined the village residents seated listening to the impromptu performance. Before putting my recording equipment away I asked Balikoowa about the woman and her instrument. He shrugged his shoulders saying that he was also curious because he had never heard "a lady *akadongo* player." Vilimina Nakiranda introduced herself as the leader of the local Bakuseka Majja Women's Group and asked if we would also like to record *her* and her songs. As she accompanied herself, Vilimina sang a powerful series of songs in which she outlined ways women must fight back against AIDS, reclaim their health, and change their lives—Vilimina was in fact *singing for life!*

Music is a powerful tool used today by women and youths in many areas of Uganda—rural and urban. Studies of HIV/AIDS and musical performances in Africa are urgently needed in order to help guide and direct funding agencies, relief workers, educators, and local non-governmental organizations concerning the power of localized forms of disseminating information. Women's indemnity or social groups in eastern Uganda fight an uphill battle on a daily basis against a fast-spreading disease, and for many already infected with HIV, time is running out. Women sing, dance, and perform dramas during their group gatherings to introduce interventions that focus on gender issues specific to women and female youths; many song texts warn against participating in risky environments or engaging in unprotected sexual behavior. Many songs also outline support networks available from the greater community (including the availability of condoms and testing). Music is used by many of these groups to disseminate information, mobilize resources, and raise consciousness concerning issues related to HIV/AIDS. I believe that the critical responses by women in the form of musical performance should be understood as a significant means of constructing practical approaches to HIV/AIDS prevention and education.

Women's Groups: Toward a Medical Ethnomusicology

The chance meeting with Vilimina outlined above has opened many opportunities for me over the past four years to record, interview, interact with, and get to know women who gather in order to educate other women and discuss issues related to HIV/AIDS testing, care, treatment, and counseling in Uganda. This is not an uncommon phenomenon in East Africa; such social groups are frequently formed and they function in many ways as extended families, serving financial, educational, spiritual, familial, and advisory roles, and they are frequently formed by women in both villages and cities. That many of these contemporary women's groups in Uganda, such as the Bakuseka Majja Women's Group, turn to

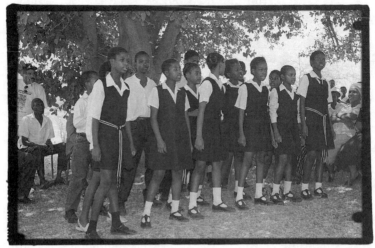

Courtesy of World Vision

musical performance—songs, dances, and dramas—to increase the understanding of reproductive health and female sexuality, and to promote the adoption of safer sex practices, is not unusual in this area of the world, and there is a great (and urgent) need for documentation and further analysis and compassionate understanding of this performance tradition.

Uganda has historically been at the very center of the HIV/AIDS pandemic, in terms of the global conscience and regarding local funding of research on the control and monitoring of fluctuations in infection rates. Testing, education, awareness, and treatment have become highly politicized as demonstrated in President Museveni's initiative to treat the virus and disease as an "open secret"; in this regard the country has dealt aggressively with HIV/AIDS to a much greater extent than other countries in sub-Saharan Africa. According to latest figures from the Center for Disease Control, more than 400,000 people have died from the disease since first diagnosed in the country in 1984; yet another two million people are now infected with the virus. At one time, these figures represented approximately 30 percent of Uganda's total population; current infection rates are reported to be under

8 percent. The HIV infection rate in Uganda is estimated as high as one out of four in the eastern villages where young women are facing phenomenal risks of HIV infection and ultimately death from AIDS.

Yet by listening to women's voices we have an opportunity to move beyond charts and diagrams, figures and statistics, to refocus attention on how grassroots efforts to educate and affect change are having significant effects; the musical performances of many women's groups now complement and in some cases are integrated into the efforts of local governments and private and multinational and bilateral non-governmental organizations to combat the disease. The field research I engage with women's groups in Uganda is one of the first to focus on what might be termed "Medical Ethnomusicology," since it directly relates to issues of disease, suffering, bereavement, health care, and related topics.

Music, Dance, and Drama as Medical Intervention

No one will listen to us *unless we bring our drums!*
No one will listen to us *talk* about *Silimu*—AIDS—*unless we dance!*

I sit in a small family compound in Bute Village in the Busoga region of eastern Uganda surrounded by banana trees, fields of cassava, and a dwindling coffee crop. I am struck by the statement about drums made by Aida Namulinda, a farmer, and leader of the local village women's music and dance ensemble with whom I have come to work. Two medical doctors accompany me and Alex Muganzi Muganga and Peter Mudiopeæboth of whom are involved with HIV/AIDS medical research in Kampala, the nation's capital. While the doctors and I set up our recording equipment, Aida continues to mobilize her village's performing ensemble in order for our research team to document several of the group's songs, dramas, and dances.

As the evening-long music making begins, several men bring out a set of *kisoga* xylophones, panpipes, tube fiddles, and drums from

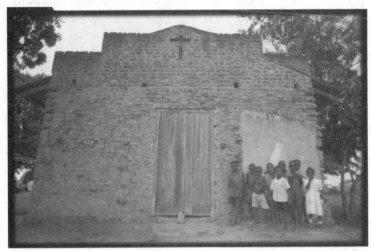

Courtesy of Jonathan W. Rodgers

one of the huts to accompany the women of Aida's group as they summon and engage the community of farmers returning from the fields. The women encourage everyone gathered to dance, sing, *and listen to the group's messages* concerning proper condom use, faithfulness to partners, and sexual abstinence.

During a break, Aida continues her thoughts about music with me, asserting that whether by itself or incorporated within dance and drama, music is now embraced by village-based groups such as hers as the most effective and immediate means available for communicating, educating, and disseminating information pertaining to medical and health care concerns. As she returns to lead the group of women, Aida dramatizes a powerful series of songs outlining specific ways women can fight back against the *spread* of HIV/AIDS, and how they must reclaim their health and change their lives even though they are all HIV positive.

Aida—and many other women in Ugandan villages and towns—use music, dance, and drama more than ever to engage aggressively the devastation the HIV virus has caused in their communities. In many of these communities women now often raise multiple generations of orphaned children while simultaneously planning for the inevitable need for similar care and education for their own offspring. With little—and often times no—support from governmental agencies and local and foreign non-governmental organizations (NGOs), women's indemnity groups now often turn to more traditional and demonstratively more effective means of communicating *information* in traditional Ugandan culture—*music, dance,* and *drama*—for purposes of healing, counseling, care, and education . . .

Musical Performance

Most groups with whom I have worked compose their own songs and dramas, drawing on *local* musical and dance traditions to support and anchor their performances. None claim to have "borrowed" their mate-

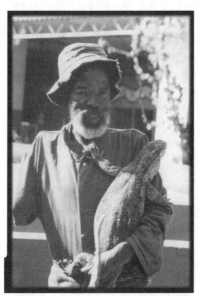

rials, although several groups have songs in their repertoire that originate with music and drama groups such as TASO, the AIDS Support Organization in Kampala—songs such as "When We Lose One Member" are common to several groups. The didactic efforts of women's group are typically located within traditional performance contexts. Several village groups draw on traditional forms of dance, drama, and music to demonstrate the problems that can arise if one turns solely to

Courtesy of Pam Kidd the traditional, local medical model—the witchdoctor—rather than embracing the so-called Western medical model.

Women's indemnity groups in eastern Uganda fight an uphill battle on a daily basis against a fast-spreading virus and disease. Many such groups sing and dance for themselves and for others to introduce interventions that focus on gender issues specific to women and female youths, and their songs and dramas warn against participating in risky environments or engaging in unprotected sexual behavior. These village performances also outline support networks available from the greater community (the availability of condoms and testing), as well as disseminating information, mobilizing resources, and raising consciousness concerning issues related to HIV/AIDS, and to counsel and support women in individual groups.

My work thus far with over forty-five women's groups (groups such as those led by Aida Namulinda and Florence Kumunu) has afforded me many opportunities to record, interview, and get to know women whose indemnity groups function as extended families—serving financial, educational, spiritual, and advisory roles. That many of these groups sing, dance, and dramatize their response to a crisis in reproductive health and female sexuality, and promote the adoption of safer sex practices is not unusual and should come as no surprise in this area of the world.

Conclusion

Drama and music groups led by women are affecting great changes, and perhaps no place greater than at the grassroots in Uganda. In many cases, the government has not been in a position to act, where women's groups working without any funding have been most successful. It was repeatedly surprising for the doctors with whom I worked that efforts to fight the virus and disease in villages were primarily in the form of musical responses and musical initiatives. On multiple occasions, they asked women *living positively with HIV* why they persisted in their efforts to contribute to local interventions, why they continued to dance when they had such little energy? The answers given remain profound: Ugandan women do not want other women and other children to experience what has been *forced* on them, and they will use whatever power they can access to introduce social and political interventions, no matter how small the reward.

This brief reflection represents at a basic level the efforts of many women and women's indemnity groups throughout Uganda to combat the HIV virus and AIDS disease in ways in which local governments and private multinational and multilateral non-governmental organizations have been largely challenged. Local and external funds have difficulty trickling down to the village networks that comprise the majority of the country. Any observations based on my field research must therefore take into account a challenge issued to me by several women's groups; this challenge is to demonstrate the *link* between the recent decline in Uganda's infection rate and the grassroots efforts of rural and women's groups. Efforts based on the Western medical model have proven largely inaccessible and expensive, and only when supported and encouraged by performances drawing on local musical traditions have medical initiatives taken root and flourished in local health care systems.

PAUL O'NEILL

Secretary of the Treasury
of the United States of America

Speech from the Chris Hani Baragwanath Hospital, South Africa
May 24, 2002

*G*ood morning, *I'd like to welcome Secretary O'Neill and Bono and honored guests. On behalf of the Prenatal Research Unit, I'd like to thank you all for your support and your love, especially for taking your time to listen to the mothers and the HIV Research Unit and the HIV SA would like to thank you all for coming here.*

Secretary O'Neill: You know the day was made for me when we came in and we said *hello* to the people who were in the pharmacy window, and my daughter who is with me and my wife found me a baby to hold. The baby back here in the pink suit is the most beautiful baby. So this was really special.

Then we had an opportunity to spend quite a bit of time talking to the mothers. They had their babies with them, and [we heard] about their life experiences and what they have been going through and what they hope and pray for themselves and for their children.

Then we began exchanging ideas and asking for information, and I must tell you I was really heartened by the numbers we were given. I will give you some of these numbers, because it demonstrates that this problem—the treatment problem—can be financed. I asked

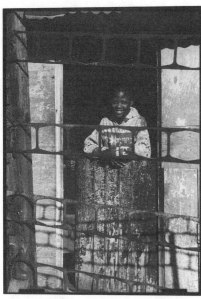

Courtesy of Recah Theodosiou

how much money is coming into South Africa last year from NGOs, and the answer is $50 million. For this nearby population in Soweto, we are talking about maybe two thousand mothers a year who need treatment, in addition to ensuring that they don't transmit their disease to their babies, either during birth or before birth. They were talking about basically $1,000. Let's say roughly $1,000. We're talking about $2 million per year.

When the NGOs are sending them $50 million—and I'm the one who is really interested in the facts—I'm saying, where is the money going if it is not going for treatment for mothers? The answer is a little elusive: it's going for prevention, and that is okay. Prevention is okay. But one of the things they teach in medical school is the idea of triage. That means you treat the most important first, not last. So for me there is an essential question when I see real people sitting here with us and know that there are thousands who are not getting any treatment. I see that there is something wrong with the allocation system if the treatment does not come first. It is not that we should not do prevention too, but there is something wrong if the system does not take care of here and now physical mothers and their babies.

So, not only do we need more money—and incidentally I want to say today that USAID is raising [its funding] from last year to this year, from $9 million to $15 million, so there is a contribution coming in that very direct way from the people on the ground here in the U.S. Agency for International Development, which can help. But we need more money. And we need better decisions about the priorities that the money is used for because the needs are so compelling.

If you just sit and talk for an hour with these wonderful people and hold their children, no one can say *no*. So we need to say *yes* together. We need dedicated people like the staff that is here—who care—to make all of this happen. I agree with you. Our resolve should be to send you back to the well-baby clinics.

Thank you all very much.

This speech is in the public domain.

NOELINA NAKUMISA

Director of Meeting Point

Meeting Point:
Dignity, Value, and a Certain Degree of Humanity

We have over 850 adults and children who do not have anywhere to stay, who do not have anything to eat, who have nothing to wear, and who, of course, do not have any medical care.

Meeting Point, a small non-governmental organization in Kampala, Uganda, was a product of the experiences of a group of friends who found themselves confronting the HIV/AIDS problem *in every aspect of their lives*—either from being personally infected, from caring for someone within their family, or helping with the care of a dear friend. My friends desired to dig deeper into their own lives and the lives of their neighbors in order to discover the very meaning of suffering and death. Our initial goal was to establish a social system whereby our families and friends would no longer be abandoned when it was determined that they were infected and affected by HIV/AIDS.

Many families in Uganda—as in other parts of Africa—have been broken up. Denial, fear, and suspicion can quickly enter into relationships between husbands and wives, parents and children, when HIV/AIDS enters a social system. A major problem today is that we typically do not (perhaps because we cannot) have the ability to love our very own lives. If we cannot begin to look at each other and treat each other as human beings, as persons, then we fall into the trap of "using" each other as things, as animals, or according to our own needs

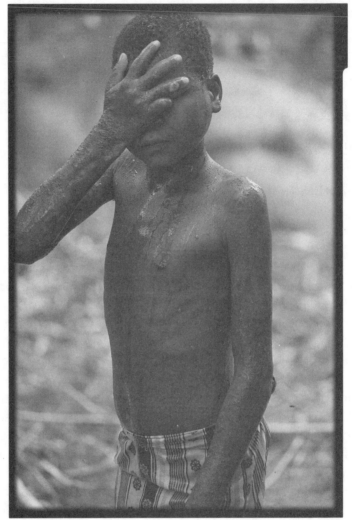

Courtesy of World Vision

and instincts, and when we are not satisfied we may become violent with others and even ourselves. Condoms and fear are negative measures that conflict with our ability to practice self-love. The problem of HIV/AIDS is one of the major problems of our lives in Africa. It is a problem of our very humanity, provoking and awakening in us a discovery of the full dignity and value of human life and love.

At Meeting Point we offer counseling to patients with HIV, lessons in behavior change to all youth, adults, orphans, and their families. We provide health education and counseling on various sexual behaviors. We also engage home visits to patients, orphans, and infected-affected families. We do our best to provide medical support to those who cannot afford to pay their hospital bills, and we give advice on hygiene or facilitate help in cleaning the houses of those too weak to clean by themselves. The volunteers at *Meeting Point Kampala* distribute food and domestic kits to those in need and provide some payments of rent to those who have been abandoned. We support the school fees of orphans at least for the primary level of education and try to track the progress of malnourished children and their mothers, educating mothers on ways to feed their children and themselves. Recently we have focused considerable attention on social concerns such as legal problems experienced by our clients: many widows, patients, and orphans, for example, are unable to inherit under current laws. To those who specifically request it, we seek out ways of providing religious instructions, to enable them to receive particular sacraments.

In all our activities, our primary goal is to restore a certain degree of humanity, that real sense of individual humanity, because when someone discovers the meaning of his or her individual humanity they discover individual and infinite dignity and approach new ways to find value in their lives. Our goals are simple and holistic. We strive to care for totality of the lives of AIDS patients and orphans, not for any one particular aspect of their lives. A main objective of our work then is to create a true relationship, to make friends out of clients.

AIDS in Uganda

In spite of real progress in promoting human development, Uganda is still ranked among the poorest countries in the world. Societal indicators such as per capita income, infant mortality rate, primary school enrollment, and general life expectancy locate it among one of the weakest in East Africa. The prevalence of HIV/AIDS has affected the once productive labor force through overwhelming death. Current estimates suggest that about 1.9 million Ugandans now live with HIV/AIDS. Approximately 70 percent of documented cases are in the most productive age—that is between fifteen to forty-five years old—and girls are six times more likely to be affected than their male counterparts.

We are a particularly vulnerable country in the plight of poverty and AIDS. The impact of HIV/AIDS on women in particular affects their position as producers of food and caretakers of sick family members and orphans. Moreover, women have a very low level of education and high illiteracy rate that makes it even more difficult for them to secure employment or benefits from technological advances. The Ugandan government has, however, recently adopted a progressive gender and development policy that specifically promotes women's economic and political empowerment. At the same time, the Ugandan government fully recognizes that HIV/AIDS poses a real and serious threat to overall socio-economic life and development. For this reason it has established key policy guidelines for HIV/AIDS control through a multi-sectoral approach that includes all the social partners involved in the process.

Children and AIDS in Uganda

Children are the second principal group most vulnerable to and affected by poverty and AIDS. It is estimated that there are 1.7 million orphans living in Uganda (estimate as of June 2000), most of them orphaned due to the AIDS epidemic and civil strife. Many of these orphans have also become street children, living in the streets, far away from their extended families, alone or in groups of other children.

Meeting Point has begun to care for street children and their everyday needs, and in particular those who are orphaned by HIV/AIDS in the Namuwongo area, just five kilometers from Kampala the capital city of Uganda. Namuwongo is a slum area where the living conditions of the people are extremely poor and the immunity of the people to infections is very low. AIDS is as common as malaria and an increasing number of orphans and patients have been abandoned there with no place to stay.

In 2000, Meeting Point established a basic education program benefiting children—especially girls, aged ten to fifteen years old—who never had access to formal education. There are currently two hundred children enrolled in the Learning Centre which provides basic education, music, dance and drama instruction, catechism, formal and informal education, first aid, handcrafts skills and general knowledge, especially regarding hygiene and behavior change. The Learning Centre is located in timber hall and has been successful in raising funds to send children to formal primary schools. At the Centre children are taught issues related to behavior change, which turns them into better, more knowledgeable adults. They learn to read and write and learn handicraft skills, which results in an important stable source of income. Some children who are above the primary level age are taken to Vocational Schools for further training.

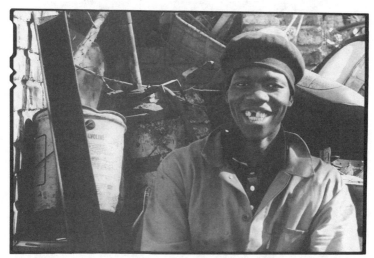

Courtesy of Recah Theodosiou

Meeting Point Vocational Training

Training in vocational skills is offered specifically to girls with different backgrounds, many of whom are unable to continue with formal education due to a number of reasons, e.g. losing their parents and nobody can help them continue with their studies, becoming mothers at an early age due to sexual harassment, poverty, or customary attitudes. Through vocational training, basic education, and

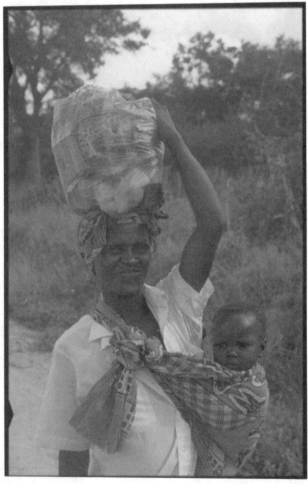

Courtesy of Pam Kidd

recreational activities, the skills of adolescent girls have been greatly developed with the goal of helping them to support themselves and their families since the majority of young girls now live in child-headed families. Since 1999, sixty-two adolescents have benefited from this program, which offers tailoring skills, handicrafts, and adult literacy classes. Twelve girls are already earning a living in tailoring and others are doing different jobs. In addition to this, they are given contracts from the offices of Meeting Point to make uniforms for sponsored children from different schools as well as people from outside.

Kyamusa Obwongo Women's Group

The women's groups at Meeting Point attempt to communicate issues related to behavioral change through programs drawing on local music, dance, and drama. Educational messages have helped change the lifestyles of people in our community most especially by encouraging and enabling people who are HIV negative to remain so. In addition, many AIDS patients gain the courage to go public in order to advise others to reduce the spread of AIDS and ways in which to live positively. This has set a good example in our disadvantaged community by promoting safer sexual behavior and by enabling people to live more happily during the last days of their lives. Members of the women's group are also able to access loans from a revolving fund which currently has 120 members, each with an average of eight people in a family—that is to say that at least 960 people have benefited in this loan cycle.

Music Dance and Drama

Since we now know that AIDS is a preventable disease and that much of the prevention lies in education and consequent behavior change, Meeting Point chooses to pass all messages about AIDS, poverty, and ignorance through the arts in order to best sensitize the community. Our main messages are communicated through poems, songs, plays, and dances with the goal of reducing the rate at which the HIV virus is spread. For many infected members, music, dance, and drama contribute to living longer and more happily during the last days of their lives and helps those who are not yet infected to remain negative. Different messages to the youth and adolescents encourage them to abstain until they are mature enough to get married, avoiding free gifts from "Sugar Daddies" who can spoil their future. Since the drama group members come from different parts of Uganda, Meeting Point has a variety of traditional songs and dramas in different languages, making it easier to communicate to a wide variety of people from different ethnic groups. Education through entertaining has attracted government officials, individuals, and the community at large.

Through our reputation in AIDS education through performance, friends from Vanderbilt University in Nashville, TN, specifically Professor Gregory Barz, invited me to the United States as a representative of Meeting Point to share and educate about our joint fight—America and Uganda—against HIV/AIDS. I learned a lot from the people and agencies in Nashville, specifically regarding their loving hearts. The fact that Nashville and the rest of the world wants to learn more about Uganda's musical fight against HIV/AIDS encourages us even more to reach out across borders.

Conclusion

We have two life moments that are unparalleled in awakening a sense of awe—the miracle of birth and the miracle of death. Witnessing birth and standing in the presence of death are the only experiences where we fear that life is inherently fragile. AIDS tells the whole world to value loss and that loving carefully is not enough. We must all learn to love responsibly.

Written for The aWAKE Project.
Copyright © 2002 by Noelina Nakimusa.

AFRICA REGION: THE WORLD BANK

International Banking System

The Gathering Storm:
The Rapidly Growing HIV/AIDS Epidemic

The spread of HIV/AIDS has exceeded the worst projections by far. Nearly 34 million people in the world are currently living with HIV/AIDS, and one-third of these are young people between the ages of 10-24. The epidemic continues to grow, as 16,000 people worldwide become newly infected each day. Fourteen million adults and children have already lost their lives to this devastating disease, and the death toll rises each year (UNAIDS, 1998e). Despite these alarming figures, AIDS is still an emerging and growing epidemic.

The region most affected has been Sub-Saharan Africa (SSA). (In this document, "Africa" and "Sub-Saharan Africa" are used interchangeably.) At the end of 1998, 22.5 million people, including 1 million children, were living with HIV/AIDS in SSA, two-thirds of the worldwide total. At least 4 million Africans were nearly infected with the virus in 1998. HIV does not respect borders, and its transmission is often facilitated by subregional trade routes and other migration patterns common throughout the continent. In Botswana, Namibia, Zambia, and Zimbabwe, between 20 and 26 percent of adults are infected (UNAIDS, 1998a; Annex 2). Some countries in West and Central Africa have been less affected and have been able to maintain low and stable HIV infection rates. This is due, in part, to an early response to the threat of the epidemic in some countries, and in part because a less virulent strain (HIV-2) predominates in these countries. However, there is no single factor or clear-cut group of factors that determines the severity of a country's HIV/AIDS epidemic.

Deaths due to HIV/AIDS in Africa will soon surpass the 20 million Europeans killed by the plague epidemic of 1347-1351 (Decosas and Adrien, 1999).

It is estimated that only 10 percent of the illness and death that this epidemic will bring has been seen. The real impact on people, communities, and economies is still to come. There is no affordable cure or vaccine likely to be available in developing countries for a decade or more. The only options are to prevent further spread of the epidemic, minimize its impact, and provide a caring and compassionate environment for those infected and affected. This crisis calls for an expanded and intensified response to mobilize governments, civil society, the private sector, and the international community to take action, increase resources, and build capacity to sustain efforts to slow the spread of the epidemic.

HIV/AIDS Devestating Impact on Development

The HIV/AIDS epidemic is not only the most important public health problem affecting large parts of SSA, but also an unprecedented threat to the region's development. It is, therefore, a development crisis.

The most disturbing long-term feature of the HIV/AIDS epidemic is its impact on life expectancy, making HIV an unprecedented catastrophe in the world's history. Among 18 countries in SSA that experienced a declining or stagnating life expectancy during 1990-1995, all but one (Togo) were described as having a generalized HIV/AIDS epidemic, that is, an HIV prevalence of more than 5 percent in the adult population. Conversely, of 29 countries that experienced an improvement in life expectancy, only two, Mozambique and Lesotho, had a generalized epidemic (World Bank, 1999).

In nine African countries with adult prevalence of 10 percent or more, HIV/AIDS will erase 17 years of potential gains in life expectancy, meaning that instead of reaching 64 years, by 2010-2015 life expectancy in these countries will regress to an average of just 47 years; this represents a reversal of most development gains of the past 30 years—affecting an entire generation (UNAIDS, 1998e).

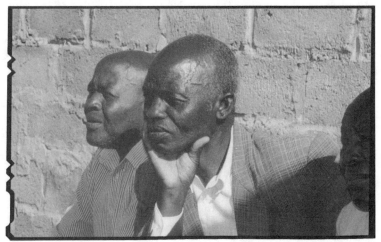

Courtesy of Pam Kidd

HIV/AIDS is also surpassing malaria as the leading cause of death in many countries.

Demographic projections vary in predicting the effects of the epidemic on population growth. However, all agree that there will be a decrease in annual population growth in the region by 2010. It is unlikely that the epidemic in any country will reach proportions severe enough and cause a rapid enough decline in fertility to exhibit a negative population growth due to HIV (Decosas and Adrien, 1999).

Child mortality is rising. In 1998, about 53,000 HIV-infected children were born in SSA, about 90 percent of the world total. By

2005-2010, infant mortality in South Africa will be 60 percent higher than it would have been without HIV/AIDS (61 deaths per 1,000 infants born rather than 38 per 1,000 in the absence of AIDS). In Zambia and Zimbabwe, 25 percent more infants are already dying than would be the case without HIV. By 2010, Zimbabwe's infant and child mortality rates will have doubles (UNAIDS, 1998e).

Young people are disproportionately affected. Worldwide, about half of all new HIV infections occur in young people ages 15-24. In 1998, nearly 3 million young people became infected with the virus, equivalent to more than five young men and women every minute of the day, everyday of the year (UNAIDS, 1998a). Girls become infected younger and die earlier than boys due to age asymmetry in sexual partnerships. In countries such as Ethiopia, Malawi, Tanzania, Zambia, and Zimbabwe, for every 15- to 19-year-old boy who is infected, there are five to six girls infected in the same age group.

The disease mainly strikes people in their prime years. Worldwide, AIDS hits people hardest in their most productive years. This profoundly disrupts the economic and social bases of families. When a family loses its primary income earner, its very survival is threatened. It sells assets and exhausts savings to pay for health care and funerals.

Children are being orphaned in huge numbers. In 1997, approximately 1.5 million children in SSA were orphaned by the disease. (UNAIDS has defined orphans as children under 15 who have lost their mother or both parents to AIDS.) To date, there are 7.8 million AIDS orphans in this region alone. In some hard-hit cities, orphans comprise 15 percent of all children (UNAIDS, 1998a). Care for these orphans often falls on extended families, stretching the capacity of these social safety nets. Many orphans are now heading households. They are far less likely to attend school, more likely

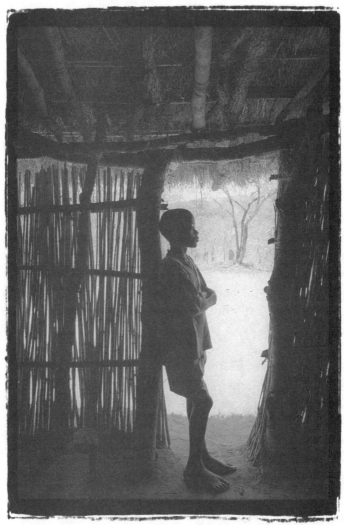

Courtesy of World Vision

to be undernourished, less likely to receive immunizations or health care, and usually very poor. Orphans often end up on the streets, where they pursue survival strategies that put them at great risk of contracting HIV themselves (USAID, 1997).

National income is affected. The illness and impending death of up to 25 percent of all adults in some countries will have an enormous impact on national productivity and earnings. Labor productivity is likely to drop, the benefits of education will be lost, and resources that would have been used for investments will be used for health care, orphan care, and funerals. Savings rates will decline, and the loss of human capital will affect production and the quality of life for years to come. Countries need to plan for the human resource needs that will result from the millions of premature deaths.

The epidemic is having a tremendous subregional impact. Southern Africa has one of the world's most rapidly spreading HIV/AIDS epidemics. The eight countries with the highest prevalence rates in the world . . . ranging from 12 to 25 percent of the adult population, are in Southern Africa. Zimbabwe is especially hard hit with up to 50 percent of pregnant women in some sites infected. In Botswana, Namibia, and Zambia, the prevalence rates among pregnant women are between 20 and 40 percent. South Africa trailed behind many of its neighbors in 1990 but is rapidly catching up. In 1998, South Africa accounted for over half of all new infections in Southern Africa and for one in seven new infections in SSA. The socioeconomic costs of South Africa's HIV/AIDS epidemic are critical not just within the country itself, but for its neighbors as well, given the interconnectedness of many economies to the economy of South Africa and the high degree of movement among countries in the subregion.

The Imperative of Urgent Action

The cost of inaction. Although prevention strategies were known early in the course of the epidemic and many interventions have been implemented on a limited scale, only a few countries have taken sufficient action to curtail the spread of HIV/AIDS. Inaction to date has resulted in millions of new infections and unnecessary deaths, leading to the current crisis situation that will require considerable effort and resources to bring the epidemic under control.

In 1982, there was only one country in Africa, Uganda, with an adult HIV prevalence rate higher than 2 percent. Today there are 21 countries in Africa with prevalence rates of more than 7 percent. Since 1985, the prevalence of HIV in urban antenatal women in Blantyre, Malawi, has increased from less than 5 percent to over 30 percent. In Francistown, Botswana, reported rates in antenatal women were less than 10 percent as recently as 1991 but rose to 43 percent in 1997 (U.S. Bureau of the Census, 1998). In Ethiopia, the proportion of adults infected with HIV increased from less than 1 percent to nearly 10 percent between 1987 and 1997. These alarming figures illustrate how quickly the epidemic can spread out of control.

The cost of delaying an intensified response is monumental. More than 4 million people in SSA were newly infected in 1998, and the numbers are certain to grow in 1999. Most of these people will die within the next decade, leaving millions of orphans. The resulting social decay and breakdown will threaten socioeconomic development for decades to come.

The benefit of action. Despite the mounting crisis, the situation is far from hopeless. Although HIV prevalence rates are high, more than 200 million adults in Africa are not yet infected. However, many are vulnerable and will be infected and die unless action is taken now.

Studies have shown that specific interventions using voluntary counseling and testing (VCT), condom social marketing, peer education, and treatment of sexually transmitted infections (STI's) can change behaviors and reduce the risk of HIV. Modeling has shown that the syngergistic effect of combining these interventions reduces the risks even further. The following pilot projects were carefully evaluated and demonstrate the effect these specific interventions can have on changing behavior and reducing transmissions of STIs, including HIV:

- Results of a Rwandan study on the impact of preventative counseling and testing indicated that for women whose partners were also tested and counseled, the annual incidence of new HIV infections decreased from 4.1 percent to 1.8 percent. Among women who were HIV-positive, the prevalence of gonorrhea decreased from 13 percent to 6 percent, with the greatest reduction in those using condoms (Allen and others, 1992). The estimated costs of VCT programs in SSA is US $4.40 per person counseled and tested. (The cost estimates provided in these examples are not specific to these studies but were compiled from the literature on costs of interventions throughout SSA and represent a medium-cost scenario; Kmaranayake and Watts, 1999).

- Studies in Mwanza, Tanzania, show that early, continuous treatment of STIs in rural community was associated with a 42 percent decline in newly acquired HIV infections at a cost of US$10 per person treated (Grosskurth and others, 1995). More recent evidence indicates that STI control may be most effective in the early phase of an HIV epidemic (Wawer and others, 1999).

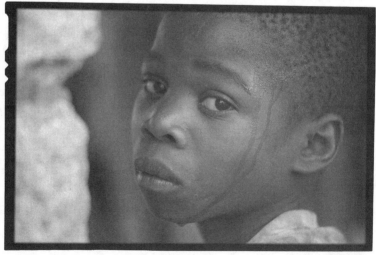

Courtesy of World Vision

The challenge is to incorporate these and other effective interventions into a comprehensive national program, bring them to scale, and sustain them. By so doing, certain countries have been able to slow the epidemic and minimize its impact. These countries have been able to change social norms to help people lower their risk of HIV and have significantly reduced the number of new infections. The active response and success of HIV-prevention efforts in these countries provide reason for hope:

- There were significant decreases in HIV prevalence among women attending prenatal clinics in certain regions of Uganda between 1990-1993 and 1994-1995. These were noted particularly among women ages 15-24 (Wawer and others, 1999). Strong, high-level national leadership and effective partnerships with civil society facilitated the changes leading to this decrease.

- The leadership of Senegal chose not to deny the existence of the epidemic, but to face the challenge from the start. Enlisting all key actors as allies in a timely and aggressive prevention campaign has helped the country maintain one of the lowest HIV-infection rates in SSA (1.77 percent). The small number of HIV-positive individuals allows the government to consider utilizing treatment schedules that otherwise would not have been affordable (UNAIDS, 1998e).

- Numerous Western countries have established and sustained comprehensive HIV/AID-prevention efforts that have greatly reduced the spread of the epidemic. The most notable features of the spread of the Australian response to HIV/AIDS are support from all political parties and strong partnerships among community groups, government officials, health workers, the private sector, and researchers (National Centre in HIV Epidemiology and Clinical Research, 1997). The Swiss strategy highlights the vitality of developing strong working partnerships with people living with HIV/AIDS, local and regional officials, and nongovernmental organizations (Swiss Federal Office of Public Health, 1999). The response to HIV/AIDS in the Netherlands has been comprehensive and progressive, particularly with respect to its community-based outreach programs and partnerships with groups at increased risk of HIV infection.

VLADIMIR BERTHAUD MD, MPH, DTMH

Director, Division of Infectious Diseases, Meharry Medical College

AIDS In Africa: Epidemiology, Clinical Spectrum, and Control Interventions

Epidemiology

Since the first African AIDS cases have been reported twenty years ago, controlling this explosive epidemic has remained a major challenge: as of December 2000, AIDS had killed 17.2 million people and left thirteen million children orphans in Africa.[1] In 2001 alone, AIDS killed 2.2 million more people in Africa. At the same time, there were 3.4 million incident HIV-1 cases in Africa, nearly 70 percent of the global total. Although it contains only 10 percent of the world population, sub-Saharan Africa shares approximately 70 percent of the forty million worldwide HIV-1 cases.[2] Estimates of HIV-1 prevalence in Africa where the epidemic is largely heterosexually driven are usually derived from surveillance tests performed among pregnant women attending antenatal clinics (ANC) selected as sentinel surveillance sites. This method is valid because pregnant women are fairly representative of the general population but it may not be totally reliable where inefficient public health infrastructure provides inadequate access to prenatal and natal care. However, in countries where the HIV-1 epidemic concentrates in a few groups with high-risk behavior, commercial sex workers and their clients, men who have sex with men, and injection drug users the methodological approach is different. In such circumstances, estimates of HIV-1 prevalence are based on prevalence in specific high-risk behavior groups and the estimated size of these populations. Since the latter are often marginalized and face many complex cultural barriers, social taboos, misconceptions, and sometimes are impeded by their own denial or HIV unawareness, they tend to be harder to reach and test. Thus, the HIV-1 prevalence rate in such populations could also be underestimated. According to the U.S. Census Bureau database, HIV-1 prevalence among pregnant women in 2001 was quite variable as shown in table 1.

Table1: HIV-1 PREVALENCE (%) AMONG PREGNANT WOMEN IN SELECTED AFRICAN COUNTRIES

COUNTRY	SENEGAL	CAMEROON	CONGO	NIGERIA	UGANDA	KENYA	RWANDA	ZAMBIA	ZIMBABWE	S. AFRICA	BOTSWANA
Major Urban Areas	.5		.1	.2	1.25	5.3	3	.69	1.1	4.3	4.94
Ouside Urban Areas	.5	.67	.5	.3		4	.03	3	3	2.9	4.82

Of note, HIV-1 prevalence among ANC attendees outside the major urban areas in Cameroon increased from 1 percent in 1989 to 13 percent in 2000 while HIV-1 prevalence among sex workers in Yaoundé increased from 5.6 percent in 1990 to 45.3 percent in 1993.

Between 9 to 17 percent of truck drivers studied in 1993-1994 were tested HIV-positive while 15 percent of military personnel was also found positive in 1996. In the meantime, HIV-1 prevalence among commercial sex workers and Sexually Transmitted Infections (STI) clinics patients in South Africa was estimated at 50.3 and 57.15 percent respectively. Sub-Saharan Africa contains the countries with the highest HIV-1 prevalence in the world: Botswana (38.8 percent), Zimbabwe (33.7 percent), Swaziland (33.4 percent), Namibia (22.5 percent), Zambia (21.5 percent), and South Africa (20 percent).

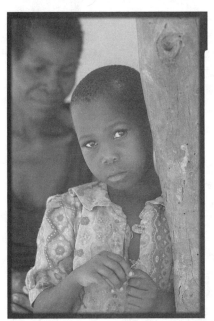
Courtesy of World Vision

Factors associated with HIV/AIDS transmission in sub-Saharan Africa have been described elsewhere: male dominance, domestic violence, rape, poverty and decline of social services, scarcity of sex education and HIV counseling and testing, reticence to condom use, high prevalence of genital ulcer infections and other sexually transmitted infections (STI), rapid urbanization and modernization, labor migration, wars and conflicts, massive population displacements, and various forms of social practices. This list is not exhaustive! In a recent study, Gregson and colleagues have found that the substantial age difference between female and male sexual partners in rural Manicaland, Zimbabwe, is the major behavioral determinant of the more rapid rise in HIV-1 prevalence in young women than men.[3] Social and cultural systems in many African countries dictate that women have no control over their sex lives, or the sex lives of their husbands outside marriage.

Industrialization and urbanization, trade and commerce, wars and civil unrest had all contributed to increased vulnerability of women to STI and HIV transmission.

Nearly all HIV/AIDS cases in Africa are due to non-B clades while group O is primarily found in Cameroon and neighboring countries. Certain biological differences may be relevant; for example, in a cohort of 1045 adults in Uganda, subtype D is associated with faster progression to death (relative risk 1.29) and with a lower CD4 cell count compared to subtype A.[4] A sequential and phylogenetic analysis of the reverse transcriptase region of five HIV-1 isolates from treatment-naïve Ethiopian émigrés to Israel discovered that variants resistant to nevirapine, delavirdine, and efavirenz were more rapidly selected at lower drug doses culture with clade C than with clade B wild-type isolates. In the case of subtype C, selection with nevirapine and/or efavirenz led to the appearance of several previously unseen mutations in reverse transcriptase region as well as other previously reported mutations.[5] HIV-2 occurs in epidemic form only in Africa. It is most prevalent in Guinea-Bissau, Burkina Faso, Mali, Senegal and Côte d'Ivoire. The patterns of transmission are similar to those of HIV-1 but disease progression is much slower.

The Clinical Spectrum of HIV/AIDS in Africa

As highlighted by Morgan and colleagues, in a longitudinal, prospective cohort study in rural Uganda, the presence of symptoms does not offer a reliable clue for staging HIV disease. The most common clinical conditions used to define progression of disease, i.e., weight loss, mucocutaneous manifestations, bacterial infections, chronic fever, and chronic diarrhea are also frequent in the general population. Herpes zoster, oral candidiasis, and pulmonary tuberculosis were more indicative of HIV-1 infection.[6] Thus, the routine use of expensive surrogate markers tests such as CD4 lymphocyte count and HIV-1 viral load in standard practice is again valid. A prospective study of HIV-1 seroconverters blood donors in Abidjan discovered all but two patients asymptomatic at baseline, with a median

CD4+ cell count of 527/mm³, a median plasma HIV-RNA level of 4.6 log 10 copies/ml. During the first three years of follow-up, there were few clinical events, the median CD4+ cell count declined by 20 to 25/mm³, and the median plasma viral load varied very little.[7] In another prospective, longitudinal study in rural Uganda, the median time from seroconversion to AIDS was 9.4 years, and from AIDS to death 9.2 months.[8]

Gastrointestinal disease, mucocutaneous manifestations, septicemia, cryptococcal meningitis, and pulmonary syndromes dominate the clinical pattern of AIDS in Africa. Chronic diarrhea and wasting are frequent characteristics of AIDS in Africa. *Cryptosporidium, salmonella, shigella, giardia,* and *Entameba* are the commonest infectious etiologies.[9, 10] Epidemic Kaposi's sarcoma is a well-characterized HIV-1 related dermatological complication. A maculopapular intensely pruritic skin rash of unknown etiology

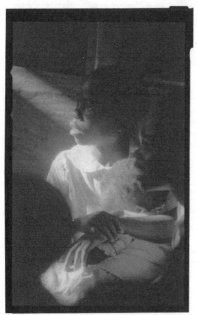

occurs most often on the extremities in a symmetric distribution.[11] This rash has a positive predictive value for HIV of 87 percent. Topical steroids and antifungal creams have not been beneficial. Severe mucocutaneous disease is a distinctive feature of HIV/AIDS in Africa. Herpes zoster is often recognized as the initial HIV-1 related illness and is more likely to present with severe pain, involvement of two or more contiguous dermatomes, a more prolonged course, bacterial superinfection, and generalized lymphadenopathy.[12] Few reports have suggested that finger clubbing may be associated with HIV infection in children and pulmonary tuberculosis in adults.[13, 14]

Courtesy of Jonathan W. Rodgers

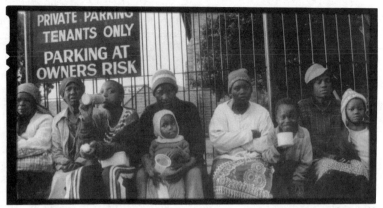

Courtesy of Pam Kidd

Life-threatening bacteremia in HIV-1 seropositive adults admitted to hospital in Nairobi is most often due to *Streptococcus pneumoniae* and multidrug-resistant *Salmonella typhimurium*.[15] In women, *Streptococcus pneumoniae* appears to cause more disease, at an earlier stage of HIV immunosuppression, than *Salmonella typhimurium* or *Mycobacterium tuberculosis*. The relative risk of invasive pneumococcal infection is 17.8 (95 percent CI 2.5 to 126.5). Pneumococcal pneumonia accounts for 56 percent of the cases.[16] Among HIV-infected patients with acute respiratory disease, bronchoscopy and bronchoalveolar lavage (BAL) identifies tuberculosis (TB) as the most common infection (75 percent), followed by bacterial pneumonia (14 percent). *Pneumocystis carinii* pneumonia (PCP) and Kaposi's sarcoma (KS) are rare.[17] However, investigation of pulmonary disease of unknown etiology in HIV-infected patients by fiber optic bronchoscopy (FOB) using both bronchoalveolar lavage and transbronchial biopsy yields different results. Nonspecific interstitial pneumonitis was diagnosed in 38 percent of the patients, cryptococcosis in 13 percent, KS in 9 percent and PCP in 5 percent.[18] We should emphasize that none of these investigators mentioned the CD4+ cell counts. In Zimbabwe, another group examined sixty-four HIV-infected patients with acute diffuse pneumonia unresponsive to penicillin and sputum smear-negative for acid-fast bacilli who underwent FOB and BAL. A much higher rate of PCP (33 percent) was found while that of TB was 39 percent. The authors reported a median CD4+ T cell count of 134/mL (range 5-355) for PCP and 206/mL (range 61-787) for TB.[19]

In Abidjan, a cross-sectional study of 2043 ambulant patients between 1989 and 1990 found that 35 percent of adult tuberculosis is attributable to HIV infection.[20] In a prospective study of 1318 women in Kigali, the two-year cumulative incidence of tuberculosis was 5.0 percent in HIV-positive women and 0.2 percent in HIV-negative women while 25 percent of HIV-positive women and 66 percent of HIV-negative women had $\geq$ 5mm induration (p < 0.001).[21] HIV infection rates in sub-Saharan African patients with tuberculosis vary from 20 percent in Kinshasa, Zaire, to 67 percent in Kampala, Uganda.[22] HIV infection impacts the clinical manifestations of tuberculosis to induce more extrapulmonary disease such as pleurisy, lymphadenopathy, pericarditis, peritonitis, and meningitis.[23, 24, 25, 26, 27] Pulmonary tuberculosis develops across a broad spectrum of HIV-related immunodeficiency. As reported from Zaire, of 216 HIV-positive patients with pulmonary TB, 32.9 percent had less than 200 CD4 lymphocytes/mL, 37 percent between 200 and 499, and 30.1 percent 500 or more.[28] However, severity of immune deficiency appears to be the major determinant of HIV-associated tuberculosis.[29] More patients seem to have fever and weight loss, produce no sputum or have negative sputum smears. Perihilar, basilar infiltrate, and miliary disease are more frequent in HIV-positive patients. Miliary TB is a common cause of hematologic abnormalities such as lymphopenia, thrombocytopenia, and leukopenia. In sputum smear-negative cases, the diagnostic yield is 86 percent for fiberoptic bronchoscopy and bone marrow biopsy, and 100 percent for liver biopsy.[30] In some African countries, *Mycobacterium tuberculosis* can be frequently isolated as a bloodstream pathogen in febrile AIDS patients.[31] Among HIV-positive TB patients, thiacetazone-containing regimens have an unacceptable therapy failure rate up to 35 percent, which is about 2.5 times higher compared with HIV-negative ones.[32, 33] This is in sharp contrast with rifampin-based therapy. In that setting, the treatment

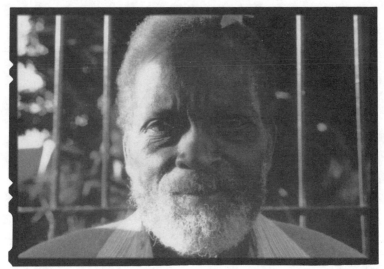

Courtesy of Pam Kidd

failure rate is similarly low regardless of HIV status (3.8 and 2.7 percent) but the higher relapse rate of 9 percent in HIV-positive patients can be reduced to 1.9 percent if the period of antituberculous treatment is extended to 12 months.[34] Twice-weekly rifampin-containing regimen administered under DOT seems to be equally curative.[35]

Control Interventions

We cannot overemphasize the importance of community outreach programs, sexual education, behavioral and lifestyle modification, empowerment of disenfranchised groups, dependable health care infrastructure, political leadership and public motivation in the fight against HIV/AIDS. An exhaustive discussion of these issues is beyond the scope of this paper. Therefore, we focus on the potential role of targeted therapeutic interventions.

I) *Control of sexually transmitted infections (STIs).* Grosskurth and colleagues had shown that improved syndromic STI treatment services in Mwanza, Tanzania, through local health units, decreased HIV-1 incidence in the general population by 38 percent. A high rate of new HIV-1 infections attributable to STIs accounts for this outcome.[36] Nonetheless, the authors of a randomized, controlled, single-masked, study of intermittent mass chemotherapy involving 12, 726 subjects in Rakai, Uganda, could not replicate those results.[37] A mature endemic, no longer concentrated in high-risk groups, is a plausible explanation. Moreover, STI intervention had no effect on the incidence of HIV-1 infection. This lends support to the priority of breaking networks of concurrent sexual partnerships early, especially between older men and young women.[38]

II) *Prevention of vertical transmission* was summarized in a recent update review article.[39] In Africa, over 95 percent of HIV-positive women lack access to combination antiretroviral therapy including protease inhibitors, depriving them of a major therapeutic option. In fact, the Pediatric AIDS Clinical Trials Group Protocol 316 (PACTG 316) and the Women and Infants Transmission Study (WITS) have reported the lowest rate of perinatal transmission of HIV-1 (1.2 percent) in cohorts of women receiving potent anti-retroviral regimens.[40, 41] Besides, the reduced rate of HIV-1 transmission with decreasing maternal HIV RNA level, and the lower resistance rate associated with the use of multiple antiretroviral agents support the Public Health Service Task Force recommendation of universal HAART among pregnant women regardless of their CD4 lymphocyte count or HIV RNA level. Unfortunately, most African women cannot afford even less complex and cheaper alternatives: short course of zidovudine, longer course of zidovudine, including intravenous infusion during labor followed by a six-week of oral zidovudine in the infant, neonatal zidovudine-lamivudine therapy, and intrapartum and neonatal treatment with nevirapine. Wherever the test is available, elective cesarean delivery at thirty-eight weeks of gestation should be offered to women with HIV RNA levels over 1000 copies per milliliter.[42] In plain reality, the majority of HIV-positive mothers in Africa are antiretroviral-naïve. Although zidovudine treatment started within forty-eight hours postpartum may be beneficial, the optimal therapy for their infants remains undetermined.[43]

III) *Prevention of opportunistic infections.* In Africa, targeted primary prevention depends on the prevalence of various opportunistic infections in a particular geographic location. Nearly across all Africa, tuberculosis is the predominant cause of morbidity and mortality among AIDS patients. Treatment of latent tuberculosis infection in HIV-positive African patients is sound and cost-effective. Acceptable regimens in order of preference include: daily isoniazid plus vitamin B6 for nine months, twice weekly isoniazid plus B6 under DOT for nine months, two-month short course treatment with either rifampin plus pyrazinamide or rifabutin plus pyrazinamide.[44, 45] In HIV-1 infected patients with tuberculosis in Abidjan, Côte d'Ivoire, a randomized controlled trial had shown that the daily administration of trimethoprim-sulphamethoxazole could decrease by nearly half the rates of death and admission to hospital.[46] In African adults at clinical stage 2 and 3 of the WHO staging system, trimethoprim-sulphamethoxazole lowered the rate of severe events leading to death by 43 percent.[47] This intervention is likely to protect against many bacterial infections such as *Streptococcus pneumoniae, Salmonella, Shigella, toxoplasmosis, isosporiasis,* and *Pneumocystis carinii.* The 23-valent pneumococcal vaccine to prevent invasive pneumococcal infection deserves serious consideration.

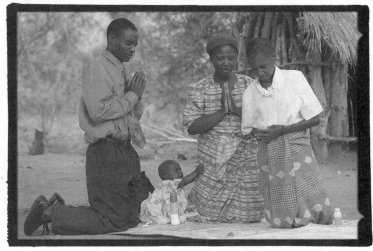

Courtesy of World Vision

At this point, there is insufficient evidence to support the routine use of fluconazole for primary prevention of cryptococcosis or histoplasmosis. In HIV/AIDS patients with presumed protozoa-related persistent diarrhea, albendazole (800 mg twice daily for two weeks) offers substantial symptomatic relief in a randomized double blind controlled trial and may be used empirically.[48]

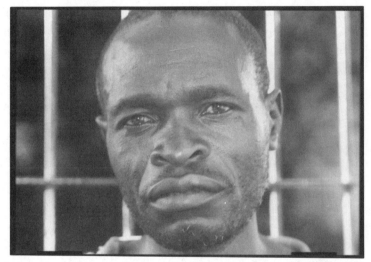

Courtesy of Pam Kidd

IV) *Antiretroviral therapy.* Resource constraint represents the stumbling block to widespread implementation of HAART in Africa. As illustrated in a paper by Guinness L and colleagues, hospitalization cost patterns for HIV-positive and HIV-negative patients at Kenyatta National Hospital in Nairobi, is similar and probably reflects the limited provision of care beyond basic clinical services.[49] A recent observational study compared the risk of tuberculosis in 264 patients who received HAART in phase III clinical trials and a prospective cohort of 770 non-HAART patients who were attending an adult HIV clinic in Cape Town, South Africa. The results suggest that HAART reduces the incidence of HIV-1 associated tuberculosis by more than 80 percent. This reduction was apparent across all strata of socioeconomic status, baseline

WHO stage, and CD4 count, except in patients with CD4 counts of more than 350 cells/mL.[50] However, we need to underscore the absence of tuberculin skin test results in this cohort and the non-integration of treatment of latent tuberculosis infection (LTBI) into the national TB control program during the study period. We should also be reminded that treatment of LTBI decreases the incidence of TB by 40 percent and might be a more interesting option in areas endemic with HIV and TB. Under the auspices of the UNAIDS HIV Drug Access Initiative, a pilot program was developed in 1997 to increase access to AIDS care and drugs in Chile, Vietnam, Côte d'Ivoire, and Uganda. An assessment of this program in Uganda showed that the combined effect of therapy, loss to follow-up, and death for all patients resulted in the probability of patients remaining alive and on antiretroviral therapy at one year close to 50 percent. This program demonstrated the feasibility of expanding access to antiretroviral drugs in Uganda and could be replicated in other African countries.[51]

Conclusion

Amidst this escalating pandemic, there is room for a few encouraging statistics. In fact, a recent study confirmed the downward trend in the prevalence and incidence of HIV-1 infection in Uganda, between January 1990 and December 1999. During that period, the incidence of HIV-1 fell from 8.2 to 5.2 per 1000 person years at risk.[52] Well-supported social and behavioral interventions account in large part for this success: increases in age of first sex for women, decreases in the number of sexual partners, increases in age at marriage for women, and delayed age of first birth. Investigators in Zambia have also reported a significant reduction in HIV-1 prevalence in women aged 15-24, from 16 percent to 12 percent during four years. Low and stable HIV infection rates have also been reported from Senegal. Notwithstanding these accomplishments, a safe, effective and accessible preventive vaccine remains our best long-term hope for the control of the HIV/AIDS pandemic. An increasing number of HIV vaccines are being developed for Africa.[53] An ideal vaccine will be one that can protect against genetically diverse HIV-1 strains. But can we afford prevention without treatment? "Health care is a human right that extends to all people, including those who are HIV positive".[54]

Written for The aWAKE Project.
Copyright © 2002 by Dr. Vladimir Bertaud.

JOHN M. WALIGGO

Professor at the Catholic Higher Institute of East Africa

African Christology in a Situation of Suffering

Theology, in all its branches, can best be understood when it is fully inserted into the cultures, times, circumstances, and concrete situations of a particular people. As the emerging theologies are trying to show, the main sources of theology include not only the Scriptures and church tradition but also the very people of each epoch with all their hopes and aspirations, their anguish and suffering.[1]

This essay tries to respond to the question: Who is Christ to the suffering people of Africa? From this central question we can derive three others: What image of Christ do the suffering people of Africa have? What image of Christ have the Christian churches and preachers presented to the suffering people of Africa? What should be the ideal and most relevant image of Christ to the contemporary suffering people of Africa? These questions are not at the periphery but at the center of meaningful christology, for as Monica Hellwig asserts: the first and all-inclusive question that Christians must ask and answer about Jesus is: What difference does Jesus make?[2]

Indeed what difference does Jesus make in the lives of the suffering people of Africa? What does faith in Jesus Christ bring to their suffering? What does *following*[3] Christ concretely mean within the African situation?

In attempting to answer the central question, five sources will be used: the present reality of suffering in Africa, aspects of historical Christian theology in Africa, biblical exegesis from an African perspective, the comparative studies of a few christological contemporary approaches and responses[4] of theological students to the theme studied.

Since the bisecting of Christian theology into quasi-autonomous branches has been a Western phenomenon, there is no intention in this paper to strictly follow the real divisions in theology. While Jesus Christ is the center of our reflection, God the father, the Holy Spirit, and the Trinity as a whole will be prominently featured as the discussion warrants. This approach is one of the ways of building a truly African theology which is not defined at the beginning but rather which naturally evolves as African theological thinking goes on.

Nature of Suffering

Suffering, as experience shows us, respects no age or condition, no place or human being. It is a reality which is ubiquitous. Only the causes, intensity, extent, duration, and attitude may differ.

For the sake of clarity, but at the risk of sounding a bit simplistic, I wish to place suffering under five categories. The first two categories should be constantly fought against in our lives and society, while the last three types ought to be positively and dynamically accepted and utilized as means to our growth to Christian maturity and to authentic and total human liberation.

Self-Inflicted Suffering. Much of the suffering we experience in and around us is self-inflicted. Through sin, misbehavior, ignorance, lack of self-control, laziness, narrowmindedness, and malice we inflict suffering on ourselves. A teenage girl who stubbornly refuses to take heed of her parents' advice against premarital sex may one day find herself suffering because of the "unwanted" and "unplanned for" pregnancy. From this single instance of self-inflicted suffering her entire life may become one vicious cycle of suffering. Several years later, this person may forget she was the original cause of her own suffering and may refer to God as the source of all her suffering.

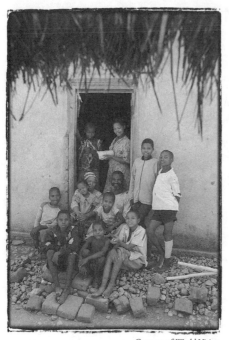

Courtesy of World Vision

Self-inflicted suffering gives birth to many "if people." Such people live always to regret, but when it is already too late. It is to this self-inflicted suffering that much of classical christology was concentrated. It is a christology founded on the main message of Christ's preaching namely, conversion. It emphasizes God's kindness and compassion. He is slow to anger and full of mercy. It is the christology of the parable of the prodigal son. It calls people to repentance and total conversion. In this christology, personal and individual sin is indeed the real cause of all evil and all suffering in the world. Against this claim, Monica Hellwig explains that:

> [I]t is at this junction that the plea arises, mainly from Third World Liberation theologians, for a soteriology and Christology that are concerned not only with contemporary experience of believers as *interacting individuals* but with the entire range of human experience of suffering and hoping and surviving and transformation, which includes the political and economic dimensions of human life.[5]

Individual sin alone cannot explain the existence of evil and of suffering in the world.

Suffering Caused By Others. Much of the suffering we witness in the world at large and Africa in particular is inflicted on the innocent people by a few selfish individuals or groups or societies of people. In South Africa, a white minority which claims even to be "Christian" continues to support and use apartheid to humiliate, oppress, rob, and kill the black Africans. In Ethiopia, Sudan, Angola, and Mozambique, just to mention a few states, people continue to die of hunger, war, and want because of selfish leaders on either side who do not want enter into dialogue and settle the existing conflicts. In the economic sector, a relatively limited number of people are continuing to amass wealth, a privilege not in practice open to the majority. In the cultural sector certain minority groups are being oppressed by privileged groups. In the religious sphere the same reality exists. Stronger religions attempt to suppress or entirely weaken the rest. This is most evident today within contemporary Islamic fundamentalism and its commitment to a general application of Sharia law.[6] In the political arena Africa has witnessed certain cases of dictatorial rule. These have caused suffering and even death to many helpless people.

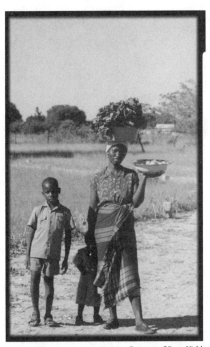

Courtesy of Pam Kidd

Classic or traditional christology has provided answers to people who suffer because of the selfishness or sins of others. These answers, however, no longer satisfy the non-Euro-American Christian world. Jon Sobrino has suggested that "basically these suspicions come down to this: For some reason it has been possible for Christians, in the name of Christ, to ignore or even contradict fundamental principles and values that were preached and acted upon by Jesus of Nazareth."[7] Sobrino adds that classic christology reduced Christ to "a sublime abstraction."[8] Christ was also reduced to a pacifist Jesus "who does not engage in prophetic denunciations, a Jesus who pronounces blessings but who does not pronounce maledictions, and a Jesus who loves all human beings but who is not clearly partial towards the poor and the oppressed."[9]

Following the same trend of thinking but arriving at a completely different conclusion, Andrew Greeley, a sociologist, is critical of the view which is quite popular today that Jesus and his message are "irrelevant" to the problems of the modern world. The irrelevance of Jesus, however, Greeley emphasizes, "is not a new discovery. He was irrelevant to his own world too; so irrelevant that it was necessary for him to be murdered. The symbolism of his life and message was no more adjusted to the fashionable religious currents of his day than it is adjusted to the fashionable religious currents of our day."[10]

Greelwy continues to explain that:

Perhaps one of the reasons for the many controversies that have raged over Jesus of Nazareth is the difficulty in classifying him. For some, he seems a simple ethical preacher; to others, a mystical prophet; to others, an eschatological visionary; to yet others, a political revolutionary; and to still others, a founder of a Church. It is not merely the different presuppositions that we bring to our study of Jesus that create the confusion. He is a hard man to categorize. He does not seem to fit into any of out neat labels, and this problem of figuring out where exactly Jesus stands is not a new one.[11]

Greeley objects to the theology of revolution on two accounts: as a social scientist and as a Christian.[12] His objection, however, seems inconsistent with his christological analysis as portrayed above. When confronted with inhuman regimes, selfish dictators who deny people their fundamental rights, racist rulers (as in South Africa), the old classic christology here would be constructed on the central theme of

Christ's message: the proclamation of God's kingdom of justice and righteousness, of peace and unity, of human dignity and universal brotherhood. This would serve as the model we use in repelling, resisting, destroying, eliminating the unjust sufferings caused by selfish or indifferent people. In such a model the theology of revolution occupies a central position. This theology is rooted in the theology of the *last resort:* when a prolonged tyranny, harmful to fundamental human values, has to be confronted by revoutionary methods.[13]

There is hardship in every endeavor to achieve a worthy goal, ambition, plan or liberation or transformation of society. The suffering involved in such hardship is only to be expected. The example of Jesus, in John 14, of the pains of childbirth for the mother is very relevant. Such pain disappears when a new child is born. It is replaced by intense joy for the mother. There is much pain in any struggle for justice, human welfare, and human dignity. The reward, however, of such struggle when it is completely or even partially won, is great joy.[14]

In accomplishing his mission of proclaiming and realizing the kingdom, it was inevitable that Christ had to suffer in order to achieve his goal. The joy he found in doing his Father's will forms a basis for a christology of this type of suffering.

Suffering On Behalf Of Others. Nothing gives as much joy to a person as to suffer in sacrifice for one he loves. To share with one who has nothing demands a sacrifice, but one which brings joy to both. To sacrifice one's entitlements for another is a highly commendable act which enriches the one who does it. Every day people make sacrifices and suffer for those they love. This may be in terms of time, goods, energy or life itself. Maximilian Kolbe who during the Second World War sacrificed his life to save the life of a fellow prisoner is a contemporary symbol of such great love. All fighters for authentic liberation of peoples, such as Mahatma Gandhi, Martin Luther King Jr., Nelson Mandela, and others, are most appealing to the contemporary Christian mind because of their option. Many mothers, in critical situations, have made an option for their children to live instead of themselves.

This is exactly what Jesus of Nazareth did. He did it in his preaching when he said: "No one can have greater love than to lay down his life for his friends" (John 15:13). He did it in action by freely accepting suffering and death, death on the cross. Whereas, therefore, the cross is a sign rejection, failure, and humiliation on one hand, it is a sign of extreme love, commitment, and liberation on the other. Since Jesus' death, many people have followed his example, giving support to this christology of extreme love which is tested through acceptance of suffering for a good cause.

Classic christology tends to shy from relating to Christ's death the daily deaths of men and women in sometimes justifiable struggles to liberate fellow human beings. It fails to draw out practical and concrete ways in which Christians can live and bear witness to this christology.

The Mysterious Suffering of The Innocent. The conscience of the upright and innocent is revolted when the wicked or arrogant are the happiest, most successful, and most secure (Psalm 73). Questions arise in the mind of the innocent sufferer: What good and just God could do this to me? Was it useless, then, to have kept my heart clean, to have washed my hands in innocence? (Psalms 73:13). This is the suffering described in the book of Job. It is the suffering Jesus underwent. He had done good to everyone. He had spoken well as no one had before. He had committed no sin. He prayed for and loved his enemies and taught his followers to do the same. Why then the passion and the Cross?

The suffering of the innocent can make the victims lose Christian faith and faith in God. The explanations given to them by some Christians resemble those given by Job's so-called friends. They add pain to pain, despair to despair. "You are suffering because of your sins, especially the hidden ones." "God is justly and openly punishing you, repent and accept your guilt." Such an approach is clearly unacceptable. Christ himself denounced it. Asked by his disciples: "Rabbi, who sinned, this man or his parents, that he should have been born blind?" Jesus' answer was brief and exact: "Neither he nor his parents sinned . . . he was born blind so that the works of God might be revealed in him" (John 9:2-3).

The type of christology for this kind of suffering which is abundant in Africa must be built on the suffering servant, in order to contribute positively to the liberation and transformation of the world.

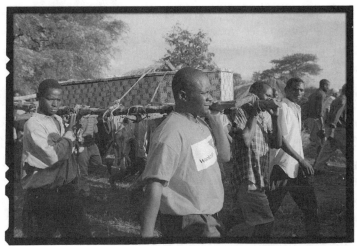

Courtesy of World Vision

Major Aspects Of Suffering In Africa.

To the outsiders, whose knowledge of Africa is obtained from the mass media, the most dramatized suffering in Africa is the lack of basic necessities of life that causes death to millions of Africans annually. These included hunger, famine, and malnutrition; insufficient and/or unclean water; lack of medicine and health care units; unsatisfactory living conditions; the large population of homeless people—the refugees, displaced peoples, orphans and widows. This type of suffering is emphasized abroad because it gives birth to compassion and stimulates humanitarian and Christian consciences to give relief to Africa. It is visible: the number of victims can be ascertained. Above all it is the type of suffering for which almost all world charitable organizations have been founded to alleviate. The philosophy, often unpronounced, which governs this approach, is to reduce the suffering without paying regard to the optimality of the structures of the societies in question.

Concentrating on this type of suffering has its advantages and disadvantages. Some victims of the above causes are assisted and saved from grim conditions and ultimately death. The virtue of sharing in concrete acts of love for a faraway neighbor in need is instilled. A glimpse of hope is given to those in despair. The disadvantages include orchestrated mass media depiction of the levels of suffering and of the generosity of the donors. For the Christians giving assistance and the Africans receiving it, the image of Christ becomes that of a grandfather who throws some sweets to the starving grandchildren, a Christ who comes in the relief "container" or in the world food aircraft or the Red Cross vehicle. Such an image of Christ is no better than that of *fac totum, deus ex machina*. In this approach there is no desire to analyze the root cause, since such an exercise would lead to greater commitment and, "worse" still, to a clear taking of sides, which international charity organizations are not prepared to do nor allowed by their constitutions.

The second aspect of suffering is in the economic sector. Poverty has given birth to much suffering. It has made the continent appear sick, crippled, and begging. This poverty is primarily caused by unbalanced economic policies which favor the already rich and powerful nations of the world. This situation was established from the time of the African slave trade, through colonialism to the present-day neo-colonialism. In the first instance the "peculiar institution" of the slave trade took away over fifty million able-bodied African men and women to develop other continents.[15] The second phase of colonialism exploited African raw materials to develop the colonizing nations.[16] Neo-colonialism has made policies and rules which dictate the wishes of the powerful over the "weak and despised" continent. All attempts to rectify this situation have failed, as UNCTAD can clearly bear witness.[17] The will to change and allow the less developed to arise is absent in the West. The present-day debt crisis is indicative of a sick world which pays lip service to the suffering majority of the world.[18]

Suffering brought by ignorance and illiteracy cannot be overemphasized. Africa has lagged behind in science and technology education. As a result most Africans cannot control or influence as profitably as possible their own environment and make it serve their needs and fulfill their aspirations.[19] In a world with so much knowledge and skills, it is a scandal that ignorance and illiteracy can be allowed to continue and dominate in Africa. From ignorance springs sufferings of disease, an inferiority complex, and feelings of helplessness.

Psychological and religious suffering in Africa is most felt in cultural oppression, racism, tribalism, and a feeling of being rejected. In this field both the colonial and missionary masters have done harm to the authentic African personality. An African Christian is a divided person, wishing to be true to both his cultural values as well as to the Gospel values—values which are often presented as opposed to each other.

Since independence, Africa has greatly suffered under the yoke of its own political leaders, many of whom adopted dictatorial approaches to government. Africa has witnessed over seventy military coups, most of which have claimed many innocent lives. There have been numerous military conflicts either internally or between the nations, giving rise to millions of refugees, widows, and orphans. Funds meant to develop Africa have been placed in personal accounts in Euro-American banks by selfish African leaders. Such leaders had neither the capacity nor the intention to propose an authentic development program for their people.[20]

Suffering in Africa is made worse through the feeling and prediction that so far there is no remedy to it; instead, suffering in all its aspects seems to multiply as years go on. The coming Third Millenium is not one of hope but rather of greater despair.[21] Despair has increased because the present situation threatens to be yet another vicious circle without a solution. As a reaction to such despair, numerous religious movements, both local and foreign, have sprung up to give assurance of *individual salvation* for the personal good of the followers.

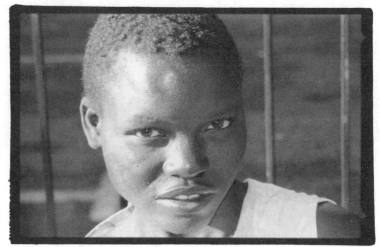

Courtesy of Pam Kidd

What Is the Root of Africa's Sufferings?

Many outsiders advance the root causes of Africa's sufferings as African tribalism, innate laziness, and lack of inventiveness or creativity. These are the easy and evident signs of Africa's backwardness to outsiders. To these, they often add corruption of the African leaders. Such people, however, fail to go a step further to ask why tribalism, why laziness and uninventiveness, and why corruption? To this category of people the redemption of Africa lies entirely in the hands of the Africans once they decide, as a community, to fight and eliminate those root causes. To me this explanation does not go deep enough.

Africans themselves are sharply divided on the root cause of their own suffering. Some advance exploitation of Africa by outsiders, an exploitation which enforces ignorance and poverty on the continent. Some suggest ignorance of science and technology which prevents Africa from competing with the developed countries. Other Africans see the root cause in the absence of total liberation of Africa and the Africans. Everywhere they argue that what can be seen is *partial* liberation which is not sufficient for the creation of the necessary attitudes and programs for integral development. The

Christian churches tend to interpret the entire suffering in a spiritualized manner which takes the presence of *sin* and the lack of *total conversion* to Christ as the root cause.

Unless there is some genuine agreement on the root cause, there cannot be an agreed-upon solution which can be undertaken with a unity of purpose.

After careful reflection, what I propose as the single root cause of Africa's suffering is *rejection*, both be

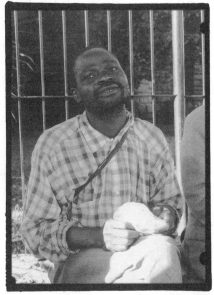

Courtesy of Pam Kidd

powerful outsiders and powerful insiders. From this rejection come all attitudes which continue to oppress Africa and intensify suffering. From rejection there comes failure to seriously think of a lasting solution to the unnecessary suffering on the continent. It is on this theme of *rejection* that my christological reflections will be constructed.

When Christianity came to Africa towards the end of the fifteenth century, its theology soon sanctioned Africa's rejection by giving support to the enslavement of Africans.[22] This created a situation which was progressively to sanction rejection of Africans in many other instances.

After almost one thousand years of isolation, when the Western missionaries came in contact with Christian Ethiopia in the early sixteenth century, they utterly rejected its Christianity as heretical and listed hundreds of errors in it. This closed the door for cooperation between the Ethiopian church and Western Christianity. When the European Christian Nonconformists were prosecuted at home, they trekked to South Africa during the seventeenth century, and on arrival they rejected the blacks, the owners of the land, as the condemned children of Ham.

The nineteenth-century theology of the missionary movement rejected any value in the African traditional religions, despised many of the people's cultural values, and would not use them as a basis for Christian evangelization.

Throughout the colonial era Christian theology rejected African church leadership. This was even the case with the Anglican Samuel Ajayi Crowther who had been consecrated Bishop in 1864 at the insistence of the farsighted secretary general of the C.M.S., Henry Venn. The rejection of his church leadership came in 1890 when many of his African pastors were dismissed without trial on fabricated accusations, and he himself was succeeded by a white missionary bishop in 1891.[23]

When nationalist movements for independence first emerged in Africa in the 1920s and more so after the Second World War, Christian theology tended to reject them as communistic and Marxist. It remained to the Catholic Portuguese missionaries in Mozambique to outright condemn as evil and sinful the African aspiration for independence as late as 1973. Christian theology, as a whole, tended to support the *status quo* of colonial rule. Once Africans succeeded in their struggle for independence, Christian theology seemed to support the neo-colonialism, the control of Africa from afar.

In the late 1960s when African theologies were emerging, they were rejected by no less a person than the scholarly Jean Cardinal Danielou in a symposium organized in Rome in December 1967. Such theologies were considered as unorthodox and opposed to the one universal theology for all.

Western Christianity has been equated to Christianity itself. Western christology has been made equivalent to Christ himself. Even today, the very word *inculturation*, is still rejected in some Western and African circles. Instances of Africa's rejection within the history of Christian theology could be multiplied indefinitely.

When all such instances of Africa's rejection by Christian outsiders and their Euro-American theology are put together, some questions arise leading to several conclusions. What is the root cause of Africa's constant rejection? For some it is the very color, black, which is the common factor uniting all Africans within the continent and those living in the Diaspora. This color, which is God-given, happened to be a sign of dirt, sin, evil, sickness, malice, and aversion according to many Euro-Americans. It, therefore, created fear, dislike, and contempt among many of them.[24] Even artistic works by Euro-Americans depicting Africans still portray an African today as clumsy-looking with huge, red lips and unproportional in size. Some rejected Africans and their continent on the basis of a biblical interpretation which in their mind represented the Africans as the condemned children of Ham, who were to be slaves forever to the descendents of Shem. Still others rejected Africa because of the many myths which were told and written about the Africans and their land. One common factor uniting all such causes is the misconception that the Euro-American world is the center of the universe. It is the model of what is good, just, and holy. It is the center of God's love and presence. As a consequence it possesses superior knowledge and wisdom, culture, and civilization, dignity and honor. When such a misconception is entertained for centuries and promoted in several ways, it becomes the heritage of the Euro-Americans. On the basis of such heritage, Africans look strange, unfamiliar, and dejected in appearance, behavior, environment, religion, and culture. Aspects of this heritage can be traced in Christian theology in relation to Africa. Missionary journals, diaries, and magazines are full of such assumptions. Christian prayer books and hymnals in Africa also show evidence of such prejudice.

It is basically such a picture and the attitudes it has generated that cause the contemporary African Christian and especially the theologians to ask themselves: Where does a church such as ours feature within the universal church? With this type of history we have gone through, what can be expected of us within the universal church? With the past attitudes of rejection still partially present within Christian theology, what should we do? What image and understanding of Christ can save us or bring us true assurance and not simply hope? As a woman theologian, Christine Reimers, recently asked: "Can a woman be saved by a male Saviour?"[25] So has one of the African people interviewed queried: "Can a white Christ accept and totally liberate the black Africans?"[26]

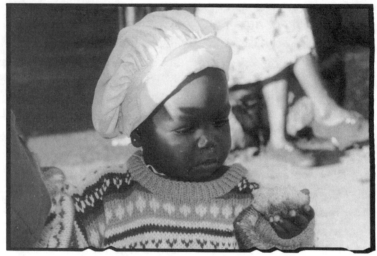

Courtesy of Pam Kidd

The perplexity and suffering of Africans would have been easier to comprehend had they come solely from the rejection by outsiders. As the post-independence history of Africa clearly shows, African have often been rejected by their own political, economic, and social rulers. Bad government in Africa has caused many deaths, forced many into refugee life, and created suffering for many people. Because of fear, self-interest, self-preservation, and sometimes ignorance, many of Africa's social, intellectual, and religious leaders have often overlooked the sufferings of their own people, allied with the rejectors, and supported the *status quo* in situations of suffering. To many ordinary African Christians, even the majority of African theologians are included among the "rejectors" of their own people. They appear to perceive that they have a monopoly of knowledge in religious and ethical matters. Instead of doing theology from and with the people and on issues of primary importance for the people, they concentrate on theological academic gimmicks which are at the periphery of people's living experience of suffering and hoping. Their theologies lack prophetic insights and witness; they lack a sense of urgency and relevance; and consequently they do not appeal to the people to whom they should minister.

Instead of succumbing to despair because of this double rejection from without and within, African Christians should look to Jesus who fully experienced rejection by the foreigners and by his own people. He certainly has something vital to say and do in the African situation and experience.

PART THREE

Engagement

How Then Shall We Pray?

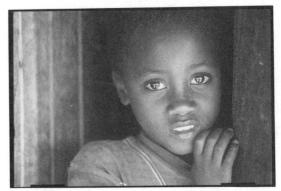

Courtesy of World Vision

A Prayer for Africa

O God, Teach us how to love, how to hope,
how to believe in Life.

We pray for healing.

We pray that you lay your hands on our brothers and sisters of Africa: the mothers, fathers, daughters, and sons. We pray that you touch their lives with your presence, your love, and your grace. We pray that you heal their hearts and minds with the gift of Life.

We pray that you heal the church. We pray that you touch the hearts, minds, and souls of all religious communities with your compelling hand of truth. We pray that you heal our fear, our anxiety, and our prejudice that we might live lives of faith, hope, and love to touch those suffering from HIV/AIDS.

We pray for salvation.

We pray that you lift up our brothers and sisters of Africa from the mire of pain, horror, and disease. We pray that you offer a gift of salvation for those who are dying, for those already dead. We pray for the living, that you bless them with Hope in the light of Love.

We pray for doctors, nurses, caregivers, and researchers. We pray that you offer them wisdom, compassion, and faith. We pray that you bless them with an intellect to boldly imagine a world without AIDS, a vision for a new generation of medical care, and an unconditional love for those who are dying without a hope for treatment.

We pray for support.

We pray that you will provide for our brothers and sisters of Africa. We pray that you will comfort them in their time of need. We pray that you will provide food for the hungry, clothes for the naked, a home for the homeless, and medical treatment for those who cannot afford such a luxury. We pray that you will provide your orphans with good families that will raise them in love.

We pray for our governments, our pharmaceutical companies, our corporations, and our religious communities. We pray that each institution finds it in their hearts and minds to offer monetary support by way of funding, medical treatments, and community-oriented aid. We pray that these institutions advance in bringing "the kingdom come, on earth as it is in heaven" by dropping the debt, providing aid, and promoting trade in Africa.

We pray for compassion.

We pray that you rain compassion on our brothers and sisters of Africa. We pray that you instill in the hearts of complacent Americans a vicarious understanding of the suffering: mentally, physically, socially, and emotionally of those dying with AIDS in Africa. We pray compassion on the cold

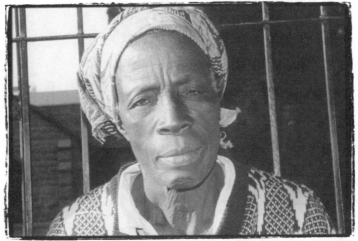

Courtesy of Pam Kidd

hearts of those who cling to ignorance and indifference. We pray for compassion on those who are compelled to combat the virus, the suffering, and the Death. We pray for compassion for the world as we attempt to wage a war against a deadly disease that is killing our brothers and sisters. We pray for compassion for Life itself.

O God, Hear our prayer.

HOW TO CORRESPOND WITH A GOVERNMENT OFFICIAL

Writing a letter is one of the most effective ways we can communicate with our elected officials. Since most representatives and senators tally public opinion to help them make decisions, think of the impact we can achieve flooding Capitol Hill with thousands of letters!

Oftentimes congressional offices equate one hand-written letter with one hundred people that support that issue. Just three to five letters to a Representative's office will force their staff to address an issue and craft a response. Your letter will make a difference!

Contrary to popular belief, it doesn't take an expert to write a good letter. Just a few sentences can convey a need and motivate our leaders to specific action. You can write a letter in ninety seconds! Just follow this simple outline:

1. Purpose first. The reason for writing should be stated in the first paragraph of the letter. State something specific and be concise. Express clearly and briefly what action you would like. One or two paragraphs should be enough. "Please make debt cancellation a priority during your term." If your letter pertains to a specific piece of legislation, identify it accordingly, e.g., House bill: H. R. _____, Senate bill: S._____.

2. Be personal. A mailed handwritten letter receives much greater attention than a preprinted card or letter. In whatever form, include your postal address. Be courteous and to the point.

3. Name the Action. Whether it is Jubilee USA Network legislation, World Bank reform or other issues, it is always good to be specific. Jubilee provides background on action issues (www.j2000usa.org) as well as on specific legislation moving through Congress. For example:
"Please vote in favor or against BILL XYZ."
"I am asking you to fully fund the debt cancellation."
"Now is the time to provide debt relief for poverty reduction in the world's poorest countries."

4. Tell why this is important. Put the situation in concrete terms. For example: "More than 18,000 children die every day as a result of international debt."
"The United States has been funding debt relief, now it is the IMF and World Bank's turn to do the same."
"Debt cancellation will renew access to safe water and primary health care and education for a billion people."

5. Address only one issue in each letter; and, if possible, keep the letter to one page.

Date
Dear Sen._____ or Rep._____,

Congratulations on your (re) election. I am writing to ask you to make debt cancellation a priority. Specifically, I urge you vote in favor of BILL XYZ that requires the United States to pressure the IMF and World Bank to cancel 100 percent of the debts of impoverished nations out of their own resources without harmful structural adjustment programs such as water privatization. Definitive debt cancellation will save the lives of over 18,000 children that die every day from debt-related causes, and transform debt into life for billions.

Sincerely,
Your name
Your address

Addressing Correspondence:

To a Senator:

The Honorable (full name)
__(Rm.#) __(name of) Senate Office Building
United States Senate
Washington, DC 20510

To a Representative:

The Honorable (full name)
__(Rm.#) __(name of) House Office Building
United States House of Representatives
Washington, DC 20515

Note: When writing to the Chair of a Committee or the Speaker of the House, it is proper to address them as:

Dear Mr. Chairman or Madam Chairwoman:
or Dear Mr. Speaker:

From http://www.j2000usa.org

Tips On Calling Your Members Of Congress

To find your representative's phone number, call the U.S. Capitol Switchboard at (202) 224-3121 and ask for your Senator's and/or Representative's office.

Remember that telephone calls are often taken by a staff member, not the member of Congress. Ask to speak with the aide who handles the debt issue.

After identifying yourself, tell the aide you would like to leave a brief message, such as: "Please tell Senator/Representative (Name) that I support/oppose (S.___/ H.R.___)."

Bill numbers for the House of Representatives start with H.R. (for House Resolution) and then the number. Bills in the Senate always start with S. (for Senate) and then the number.

You will also want to state reasons for your support or opposition to the bill. Ask for your Senator's or Representative's position on the bill. You may also request a written response to your telephone call.

Make sure to be friendly and acknowledge that the aides are handling many different issues and are often times very busy. Follow-up regularly and begin to develop a relationship with the aide that works on the debt issue. This will make a huge difference when it comes time to enlist your congressperson's support for a particular bill or action.

On E-Mailing Congress

Generally, the same guidelines apply as with writing letters to Congress. You may find and email your representatives directly from the Jubilee 2000 website. Please keep in mind that hand-written letters are far more powerful than email. Check with your congressperson's aide to find out if they like to receive emails—some offices pay more attention to emails than others.

From http://www.j2000usa.org

Visiting Your Member Of Congress

Meeting with a Member of Congress (*member* for short) or congressional staff is a very effective way to convey a message about a specific legislative issue. It is our most powerful tool to affect change in U.S. policy on debt and World Bank and IMF issues. Below are some suggestions to help you plan a powerful visit to a congressional office.

Plan Your Visit Carefully: Be clear about what it is you want to achieve; determine in advance which member or committee staff you need to meet with to achieve your purpose.

Make an Appointment: When attempting to meet with a member, contact the Appointment Secretary/Scheduler. Explain your purpose and who you represent. It is easier for congressional staff to arrange a meeting if they know what you wish to discuss and your relationship to the area or interests represented by the member.

Be Prompt and Patient: When it is time to meet with a member, be punctual and be patient. It is not uncommon for a Congressman or Congresswoman to be late, or to have a meeting interrupted, due to the member's crowded schedule. If interruptions do occur, be flexible. When the opportunity presents itself, continue your meeting with a member's staff.

Be Prepared: Whenever possible, bring to the meeting information, materials and media coverage supporting your position. Members are required to take positions on many different issues. In some instances, a member may lack important details about the pros and cons of a particular matter. It is therefore helpful to share with the member information and examples that demonstrate clearly the impact or benefits associated with a particular issue or piece of legislation.

Be Political: Members of Congress want to represent the best interests of their district or state. Wherever possible, demonstrate the connection between what you are requesting and the interests of the member's constituency. If possible, describe for the member how you or your group can be of assistance to him/her. Where it is appropriate, remember to ask for a commitment.

Be Responsive: Be prepared to answer questions or provide additional information, in the event the member expresses interest or asks questions. Follow up the meeting with a thank you letter that outlines the different points covered during the meeting, and send along any additional information and materials requested.

From http://www.j2000usa.org

HOW TO GET INVOLVED WITH EXISTING ORGANIZATIONS

These organizations are all working diligently in Africa to reduce the risk of AIDS and improve quality of life. Get involved with one or more of them today.

Africa Alive! YouthAIDS
http://www.africaalive.org/youthaids.htm

Africa Alive! YouthAIDS is a network of African youth organizations that promotes AIDS prevention and safe sexual behavior through entertainment.

African Leadership
http://www.africanleadership.org

A Christian education and development organization that trains local pastors and funds development projects in those same communities.

African Medical & Research Foundation (AMREF)
http://www.amref.org/usa.html

AMREF provides community based HIV/AIDS programs throughout eastern and southern Africa, including prevention education for high risk groups, support for income generating activities for guardians of AIDS orphans, employer-based HIV prevention programs, support for laboratory services, and training of health workers.

Africare
http://www.africare.org

Africare provides support to community-based organizations engaged in HIV/AIDS awareness, prevention and adolescent reproductive health. HIV/AIDS prevention is a component of Africare's Child Survival projects.

American Red Cross
http://www.redcross.org

In Africa and India, the American Red Cross is implementing activities under the GAP initiative in India, Malawi, and Uganda focusing on aspects of blood donor recruitment and retention, blood safety, advocacy, prevention. Home-based care activities address maintenance, counseling, drug and food provision and development of income generating activities.

American Refugee Committee (ARC)
http://www.archq.org

ARC is currently working in Africa and Southeast Asia to help control the spread of HIV/AIDS infection through training, education, and supply distribution for refugees and other vulnerable persons.

Ananda Marga Universal Relief Team (AMURT)
http://www.amurt.net

AMURT supports an HIV/AIDS program in the Nairobi slums in Kenya. They provide alternative therapies (homeopathy, naturopathy, and acupuncture) as a low-cost solution to treating symptoms, and run support groups as one small step towards creating more openness about the disease. The program also trains Kenyans as primary homeopathic health care workers.

Artists Against AIDS Worldwide
http://www.aaaw.org

Artists Against AIDS Worldwide is an entertainment and artist-led non-profit organization dedicated to raising the awareness and money needed to bring direct care to those affected by AIDS, especially in Africa.

CARE
http://www.care.org

CARE uses educational television and radio messages, offers community education programs and informal discussion groups, and trains community promoters to educate others about ways to prevent HIV/AIDS transmission. CARE also works within communities to help people living with AIDS in partnership with local health centers, ministries of health, and the private sector.

Childreach
http://www.childreach.org

Childreach, U.S. member of PLAN International, works to equip and empower community driven efforts to improve the health and well-being of children and families affected by AIDS.

Children of Promise International
http://www.promise.org

An interdenominational Christian mission organization dedicated to three areas of ministry: (1) caring for orphans and widows through church-based orphan homes, (2) reaching the unreached with the Gospel of Jesus Christ through church planting, and (3) providing for needy children through feeding and nutrition programs, free schools and higher education opportunities, and family assistance.

Christian Children's Fund (CCF)
http://www.christianchildrensfund.org

CCF works with AIDS orphans, providing them with food, health, and educational benefits (including agricultural and vocational education), as well as counseling and psychosocial support. They also teach income-generating activities so they can be self-reliant and try to identify foster care whenever possible. In addition, CCF has intervened on behalf of widows and orphaned children whose property has been confiscated by relatives of AIDS victims.

Church World Service (CWS)
http://www.churchworldservice.org

CWS is providing assistance to partners for programs including: health education and prevention; primary healthcare and treatment; sanitation and water development; and training for clergy, hospital chaplains, counselors, and Christian health professionals on dealing with HIV infections. CWS is also determining the usefulness of the Moringa oleifera tree as a nutritional supplement for persons suffering from HIV/AIDS.

DATA
http://www.datadata.org

DATA is a new non-profit organization which aims to raise awareness about the crisis of unpayable debts, the urgent need for more and better foreign development assistance, especially to fight AIDS, and the unfair trade rules which keep Africa poor and marginalized.

Direct Relief International
http://www.directrelief.org

Direct Relief International is providing pharmaceuticals and medical supplies for AIDS-related opportunistic infections to a variety of health care facilities and programs. They are also developing a special program focusing on the use of medication and baby formula to reduce mother-to-child HIV transmission.

FINCA International
http://www.villagebanking.org

In Uganda, FINCA uses their village-banking group structures as a forum for AIDS education. In addition, FINCA members have been able to qualify for group insurance rates for both health and life insurance.

Freedom from Hunger
http://www.freefromhunger.org

Freedom from Hunger's Credit with Education program combines microcredit with weekly meetings for women to learn about the virus and to develop the self-confidence they need to mobilize their communities into action. Women also learn to plan for the futures of their families if they are already infected and they develop strategies for sharing HIV/AIDS crisis information with their friends and neighbors.

Global AIDS Alliance
http://www.globalaidsalliance.org

GAA are part of a global action network working to stop AIDS through increased aid, access to medication, and debt cancellation.

Global Treatment Access Campaign
http://www.globaltreatmentaccess.org

Global Treatment Action Campaign (GTAC) is a global network for communication and organization towards access to essential medications for HIV and other diseases.

International Aid
http://www.internationalaid.org

Over the last twenty years International Aid has provided medicines, medical supplies and technical assistance to hospitals and clinics in sixteen countries of sub-Saharan Africa where HIV/AIDS is most intense.

International Center for Research on Women (ICRW)
http://www.icrw.org

Since the early 1990s, ICRW has spearheaded research on the economic and social roles of women in Africa, Asia, and Latin America that put them at special risk of HIV/AIDS infection and place on them an overwhelming burden of caring for victims.

International Relief Teams (IRT)
http://www.irteams.org

IRT pairs pregnant HIV infected women receiving ante-natal care at the hospital with mentors, HIV infected women who recently completed ante-natal care and delivered their babies.

International Youth Foundation
http://www.iyfnet.org

The International Youth Foundation and its global network of organizations working with children and youth are supporting HIV/AIDS prevention initiatives for children and youth in over twenty countries.

Jubilee 2000
http://www.j2000usa.org

Over sixty organizations including labor, churches, religious communities and institutions, AIDS activists, trade campaigners and over nine thousand individuals are active members of the Jubilee USA Network. Together we are a strong, diverse and growing network dedicated to working for a world free of debt for billions of people.

MAP International
http://www.map.org

MAP International's HIV/AIDS initiative is working to prevent the spread of HIV/AIDS in Africa and Latin America by actively engaging neighborhood churches and schools.

Near East Foundation
http://www.neareast.org

The Near East Foundation, through its health and nutrition extension program, educates people about HIV/AIDS. They especially target youth to make them aware of the seriousness and prevalence of HIV/AIDS and how to prevent it.

Operation USA
http://www.opusa.org

Operation USA enables medical clinics to function with equipment and basic primary health care supplies.

Oxfam America
http://www.oxfamamerica.org

Oxfam focuses on supporting grassroots groups coping with the societal changes brought on by the AIDS crisis.

Pact, Inc.
http://www.pactworld.org

Pact's AIDS Corps works to deepen and expand local solutions to this disease by supporting local organizations and leaders in Africa and linking them to international resources and networks.

Salvation Army World Service Office
http://www.salvationarmyusa.org

The Salvation Army's HIV/AIDS programs promote the concepts of community care and prevention. These programs provide care and support to people with HIV/AIDS and their families, and work to mobilize community resources to help people living with the disease.

Samaritan's Purse
http://www.samaritanspurse.org

Samaritan's Purse is a non-denominational evangelical Christian organization providing spiritual and physical aid to hurting people around the world.

Save the Children (SCF)
http://www.savethechildren.org

Save the Children supports community efforts in Asia and Africa to develop, implement and sustain programs for HIV/AIDS communities, including orphans and other vulnerable children.

Stop Global AIDS
http://www.stopglobalaids.org

The Campaign to Stop Global AIDS is about telling political leaders three things: donate the dollars, treat the people, and drop the debt.

The Hope for African Children Initiative
http://www.hopeforafricanchildren.org

The Hope for African Children Initiative is a community-based, pan-African effort created to address the enormous challenges faced by more the thirteen million children who have been orphaned by the AIDS pandemic in Africa and the millions more whose parents are sick or dying of AIDS-related illnesses.

The Student Global AIDS Campaign
http://www.fightglobalaids.org

Founded in the spring of 2001 to mobilize U.S. students as advocates for global AIDS, the SGAC has already built a network of students at over two hundred high schools, colleges, and graduate schools nationwide. In partnership with AIDS activists internationally, the SGAC is building a movement.

Trickle Up Program
http://www.trickleup.org

Since the mid-1990s, Trickle Up has been helping families affected by HIV/AIDS in Uganda and other African countries to start small businesses which enable the surviving children to sustain themselves after the death of their parents.

UNAIDS
http://www.unaids.org

As the leading advocate for worldwide action against HIV/AIDS, the global mission of UNAIDS is to lead, strengthen and support an expanded response to the epidemic that will: prevent the spread of HIV, provide care and support for those infected and affected by the disease, reduce the vulnerability of individuals and communities to HIV/AIDS, and alleviate the socioeconomic and human impact of the epidemic.

UNICEF
http://www.unicefusa.org

UNICEF is supporting programs that concentrate on prevention efforts among young people, especially girls, reducing the risk of mother-to-child transmission, and ensuring that children orphaned by AIDS receive health, nutritional, educational, and vocational support.

World Concern
http://www.worldconcern.org

World Concern addresses HIV/AIDS prevention through education projects. Families and communities diminished by this epidemic are supported through micro-enterprise programs. This income provides for basic needs and continues a child's education.

World Education
http://www.worlded.org/aids

Using a "training of trainers" approach, World Education programs build the knowledge and skills of government and NGO health workers, who in turn train and support community HIV counselors and home-based care providers.

World Relief
http://www.worldrelief.org

World Relief's HIV/AIDS program, Mobilizing for Life, is developing a biblically based AIDS prevention curriculum, pastoral counseling curriculum, and home care manuals to train church leaders and volunteers. Orphans are being cared for through church-centered programs such as community vegetable gardens, income-generating projects, household donations and support groups as well as microfinance.

World Vision
http://www.worldvision.org

Founded in 1950, World Vision is a Christian relief and development organization, serving the world's poorest children and families in nearly one hundred countries.

YMCA World Service
http://www.ymcaworldservice.org

Through peer education, counseling, drama, radio, advocacy, and other means, the YMCA enables youth to make positive choices for HIV/AIDS prevention and adolescent reproductive health.

How Your Community or Church Can Make a Difference

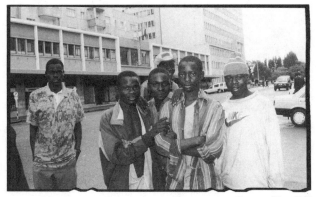

Courtesy of Pam Kidd

Your church or local community can make a tremendous impact on an African township by following one of these models below. Each outreach system helps create employment opportunities, health and quality of life improvements, and ministry outreach if desired. With a group of people working together to make a difference, you will be encouraged and sustained in your passion to help a dying continent.

HOW TO SPONSOR DRUG THERAPY FOR HIV+ MOTHERS AND THEIR NEWBORN CHILDREN

The Need. 1.6 million newborn children per year contract HIV from their infected mothers. The large majority of these mother-to-child transmissions take place in sub-Sahara Africa. Infected African newborns typically die from AIDS within three to five years.

The Solution. Nevirapine is an anti-retroviral drug that, in a single dose given at birth, reduces the mother-to-child HIV transmission rate by 50 percent. Although affordable by western standards ($.85 US per dose) it is for the most part not readily available or utilized in Christian hospitals, clinics, and community testing centers. In many countries in Africa, lack of availability is solely a matter of cost.

The Ministry Opportunity. If the evangelical church in the USA insured that every Christian-based hospital, clinic, and community-testing center in sub-Saharan Africa had access to Nevirapine we could accomplish the following goals:

- Save the lives of up to 800,000 innocent newborns each year that are needlessly infected by HIV (and subsequently die from AIDS) thus preserving a generational "remnant" of non-infected children in the hardest hit regions of sub-Sahara Africa.

- Tangibly support our fellow brothers and sisters serving on the frontlines of the HIV/AIDS battle by providing resources that will allow them to expand their ministries.

- Assist the evangelical church in North America in taking a first step of personal involvement in global HIV/AIDS ministry.

- Lay the relational foundation upon which we can build (in subsequent steps) a lasting and meaningful local church partnership to support Christian HIV/AIDS ministries in the Developing World.

The Program. Here's how a Pilot Project could work:

- Identify ten Christian-based HIV/AIDS ministries in Africa that would benefit from access to Nevirapine to reduce mother-to-child HIV transmission.

- Partner with Global Strategies (www.globalstrategies.org) to source the Nevirapine.

- A Church Relations Representative for African Leadership personally contacts mid-sized evangelical congregations in the South East, in order to find ten that are interested in participating and who will give me at least ten minutes during a Sunday morning service to present the program to the congregation.

- During the ten-minute presentation, I share four things:

  1. HIV/AIDS is a human tragedy of unfathomable proportion.

  2. In the hardest hit regions of Africa, HIV/AIDS presents the greatest opportunity for witness and evangelism in the history of the Christian church.

3. Amidst the devastation, God already has His people (like the ones I met at the Conference), who are using their own meager resources to make a difference for Christ in HIV/AIDS ministries in their own countries.

4. These called and committed fellow brothers and sisters in Christ need our help.

I invite the congregation to join with me, during the upcoming week, to *"Skip a Lunch & Save a Bunch."* We will take the money that we would each spend on one day's lunch and instead use it to buy doses of Nevirapine for use by Christian community health workers in their clinics in sub-Sahara Africa.

If 50 percent of a mid-sized evangelical congregation of one thousand gives one day's lunch money for Nevirapine, during the next year, we can save the lives of five hundred children in communities throughout the target region. That is $3.40 per life.

After placing their *Lunch Money* in the basket at the end of the service, I will ask them to pick up a *Prayer List* which will provide more information on the HIV/AIDS pandemic and the African Christian ministry that will be receiving and using their gift of Nevirapine.

I will then ask them, at some point during the next week (maybe during that lunch that we have just given up), to sit down for ten minutes with the *Prayer List* and pray for the needs and people listed on it.

Finally, if they will have me back for another ten minutes at some point in the following three months, I will return to give them a first-hand report on how God has multiplied their Lunch Money in the lives of their African brethren and the people they serve.

Prepared by J. P. Thompson and Larry Warren, African Leadership.

HOW TO SPONSOR LEADERSHIP RETREATS FOR CHRISTIAN HIV/AIDS WORKERS

The Short Term Mission Trip (SMTM) Dilemma. The dilemma of STMTs has always been *how do you insure that it is "meaningful" for both the national hosts and the visiting foreigners?* STMTs typically put a tremendous burden on the local staff and volunteers of the host ministries. In many cases, the STMT ends up being more about serving the North American visitors than assisting the host country ministries.

Again, this is perfectly understandable. Although as foreigners we mean well, we're in and out of the country in ten days or less; we don't speak the language; we don't understand the culture; and often our very presence in the community where outreach ministry is taking place is not appropriate due to the fact that we are outsiders.

Shifting the Focus of the STMT. I believe the solution to this dilemma lies in shifting the focus of the STMT. Instead of going to provide direct services to the people in the communities who are being affected by HIV/AIDS, we go instead to provide encouragement, refreshment and support for the leaders and volunteers who are actually carrying out those ministries.

North American Models. This program is modeled after *"The Cove"* (a Christian retreat run by Billy Graham Evangelistic Association); the *"Kaleo" Program* (a discipleship program for inner-city youth leaders run by Kanakuk Kamps); and *Christian Camping in the Former Soviet Union* (with Young Life).

In Step Two, North American evangelical congregations sponsor and staff a "Leadership Retreat" for African Christian workers where they can come to rest, renew, refresh and re-energize themselves for continuing HIV/AIDS ministry in their own communities.

The Program. Here's how it could work:

A consortium of up to five North American evangelical congregations (ideally located in the same metro area), who provided Nevirapine for a target region in the "Skip a Lunch & Save a Bunch" Program [see *How to Provide Drug Treatment for HIV+ Mothers and their Newborn Children*], come together to sponsor a "Leadership Retreat" for the staff and volunteers of the Christian HIV/AIDS ministries in that region.

Each congregation sends a Short Term Missions Team of at least five to eight people to staff and participate in the Retreat. Team members include a representative from the pastoral staff, missions committee, praise/worship team, prayer ministry, youth ministry, as well as a physician and several others who have proven themselves in hospitality ministries within the church.

The "Leadership Retreat" consists of an initial two-day "Homestay," where individuals on the North American Team are paired with national HIV/AIDS ministry staff or volunteers and are hosted in their homes and communities for two days and one night. During the "Homestay," team members are able to eat at their host's table, sleep in their home, go to their church and accompany them as they do HIV/AIDS-related ministry in their own community.

The goal of the "Homestay" is to expose North American Team members (in an unobtrusive way) to "the face of HIV/AIDS" in sub-Sahara Africa while personally connecting them with a

African brother or sister who is actively involved in this ministry.

At the conclusion of the "Homestay," team members and hosts, along with other regional HIV/AIDS ministry staff and volunteers reconvene at the best camp we can find, in the most beautiful area of the country, for a five to seven day "Leadership Camp."

The North American Team staffs the camp and provides the program. Pastors teach and preach; worship leaders provide the music; youth ministry leaders direct the activities and entertainment; physicians provide medical and dental care; prayer leaders direct us in times of daily intercession for our African brethren and their ministries; and the rest of us are the "work crew" who make the beds, clean the dishes, serve the food and offer the hospitality which makes our guests feel welcome and appreciated.

The goal of the Camp is to provide our African brethren with a time of spiritual, physical and emotional refreshment so that they may be energized to return to their communities, encouraged by God and by us, to carry on the valuable ministry that God has called them to.

At the conclusion of the Camp, we present each HIV/AIDS ministry represented with a monetary gift to go towards a project of their choosing.

Each North American congregation contributes $15,000 to underwrite the cost of the Homestay, the Camp, the transportation of African staff and volunteers, and a monetary gift for each Christian HIV/AIDS ministry represented. Each congregation is also responsible for the cost of their Team's travel to and from the "Leadership Retreat."

At the conclusion of the "Leadership Retreat," our African brothers and sisters go back to their communities renewed and refreshed in both their lives and ministries.

Our North American teams go back to their own churches with a broadened sense of vision, a personal connection with their African brethren, and a calling to foster their own congregation's partnership with these African HIV/AIDS ministries in more tangible and financially significant ways.

Prepared by J. P. Thompson and Larry Warren, African Leadership.

HOW TO FOSTER COMMUNITY-BASED CARE FOR AIDS ORPHANS

The Need. Africa currently has twelve million AIDS orphans, and that number will grow exponentially in the next five years totally decimating many communities, regions, and countries.

Orphans "Resonate" with North American Evangelicals. What parent hasn't shuddered at the thought of how their death would affect the lives of their children—"Who will take care of my kids, if my spouse and I were to suddenly die?" Ministry to AIDS orphans is the one ministry that will "resonate" with every parent, sitting in every pew, of every evangelical congregation in North America—regardless of whether they understand anything at all about the global HIV/AIDS pandemic.

A "Bridge" for Evangelical Church Support. The challenge of replicating community-based orphan care ministries throughout the continent of Africa can be the programmatic "bridge" which, for the first time significantly connects affluent North American evangelical congregations to Christian-based AIDS orphan ministries in the developing world.

The Program. Here's how it could work:

- Divide the USA into five target regions (NE, SE, Midwest, SW, and NW).
- Challenge up to twenty local congregations per region, who have previously sponsored a "Leadership Retreat" for Christian HIV/AIDS workers in Africa, to band together to sponsor a "City of Hope" Country Model (or community-based orphan care ministries) in a single African location.
- Sponsor congregations make an initial two-year commitment of $50,000+ per year to provide funds for supporting community-based orphan care in a designated community.

This will provide ample time to validate the program model and allow gradual transition to larger levels of government, NGO and multi-lateral organization funding for the program.

Short Term Missions Trips by members of the sponsoring congregations can provide personal involvement and assistance at all stages of "City of Hope" development—from initial construction through ongoing operations.

During the initial two-year term, continue to cultivate the sponsor church relationships in order to grow both the financial commitment and level of congregational participation in both existing and new orphan care projects.

Due to the very nature of orphan ministry, it will provide ongoing sponsorship opportunities for participating North American congregation. Potential areas for new program development include: AIDS Prevention for HIV Negative Orphans; Care for HIV Positive Orphans; Education, ESL & Job Skills Training; Micro-Enterprise Development for Income Generation; and Spiritual Evangelism, Nurture & Discipleship.

Prepared by John P. Thompson, African Leadership.

HOW TO OFFER A PASTORAL RESPONSE: PREVENTION, EDUCATION, CARE, AND COUNSELING

The Living Hope Community Center deals with the full spectrum of HIV/AIDS related needs, and develops communities in the Southern Cape Town area in order to see them change, and take responsibility for their own spiritual, physical and emotional health.

Their underlying motivation is to help fulfill the great commission by telling people the good news of the gospel, trusting that they will enter into a relationship of personal faith in our Lord, and nurturing them through discipleship into a growing relationship with Christ.

Objectives of the Project

The following objectives have been identified, based on biblical principles and problems which exist in the community:

- To spread the Good News of Jesus Christ in a life changing way, and to encourage people to follow Christ.
- To play a vital role in the prevention, care and treatment of HIV/AIDS.
- To undertake community development through educational and health related programs

How are we practically addressing this problem?

Over the past three years, many programs and projects have been developed as part of the center, in order to deal with this very human tragedy. Through these we have:

- Addressed the community lifestyle which is conducive to the spreading of HIV/AIDS.
- Addressed the spiritual needs of the community and continually are seeking to meet them.
- Targeted the children and youth with life skills programs in an effort to inculcate an abstinence based morality, thereby preventing HIV/AIDS spreading.
- Improved education at all levels:
- Provided additional education for school-going children.
- Provided adult education regarding HIV/AIDS awareness and prevention.
- Educated the community in HIV/AIDS awareness and prevention.
- Provided a center for the care of people with HIV/AIDS.
- Educated, cared for and counseled unmarried mothers, particularly those who are HIV positive.
- Provided support groups for HIV positive people.
- Offered basic primary health care, by working in co-operation with the local clinic.

Spiritual Programs

Pastoral Care—In February 2002, our first full time chaplain started at the LHCC. She leads the team of community health workers and home based caregivers, and visits and counsels the HIV positive people in there homes/shacks. Having a full time chaplain has helped greatly with spreading the Gospel, and many people have come to know Jesus through her.

HIV/AIDS Programs

Information—We offer AIDS/HIV awareness courses for community members and churches, and try to integrate AIDS awareness into all of our programs.

Counseling—We employ four community health workers who live in the community. They have a dual role in the community as care workers, and HIV/AIDS counselors who do the pre and post test counseling. Much of their work is achieved via home visiting, and they have already done well over five thousand home visits. They therefore are very important in helping us to understand the real needs within the community.

Home-based Care—We have also employed and trained up eleven home-based caregivers, who provide basic nursing care, and ambulant/palliative care for AIDS sufferers at home, as well as at the care center. The majority of our caregivers are Christians, and they play a key role in spreading the gospel in the community.

General Health Care

A massive problem in Africa is the stigmatization and rejection of HIV/AIDS sufferers. No one wants to be seen entering an AIDS clinic. Our general health care facilities are thus critically important because they provide people who suspect they are HIV positive with an opportunity to visit our premises on a non-HIV/AIDS related issue. In the privacy of the consultation they are then able to request HIV testing.

Rehabilitation and disability care—Our care-givers also carry out home visits aimed at rehabilitation and disability care.

Care center/clinic—This is run daily by a registered nurse together with the care-givers, in conjunction with the local municipal clinic. Services which we provide include wound and burns dressings, counseling, health information and non-prescriptive drug treatment. Once a week a family planning clinic is also held at the center.

Education

School—We have developed a very good relationship with the local school, and we are involved in teaching their life skills programs.

This presents with a great opportunity to educate the children and youth about HIV/AIDS prevention and awareness.

After school programs—One of the biggest problems in Masiphumelele, and many similar communities in Africa, is that the children and youth do not have much to keep them occupied beyond school. This free time leads to the opportunity of sexual promiscuity, and therefor the spread of HIV/AIDS. We have thus developed programs which take place after school in order to keep kids and young people 'off the streets'. These sessions provide:

- Extra English in the form of games and conversation
- Physical development through exercises and aerobics
- Spiritual development through devotional times and evangelistic challenges
- Social development through life skills and teamwork
- Health awareness and primary health care
- Nutritional help with sandwiches and juice

Youth Programs

As already mentioned a key aspects of dealing with this tragedy, is to provide the young people with other forms of entertainment, and this has lead to develop the following youth programs:

Coffee Bar—We are currently in the final planning stages of opening a coffee bar at the center where young people can get together and socialize in a healthy environment, which will include music, videos, and evangelistic opportunities.

Sports Evangelism—Sport is a wonderful way to entertain children and young people. We have an American basketball coach on our team who teaches and trains basket ball to the children and teenagers of Masiphumelele and other surrounding communities. Short-term mission trips of sports related evangelism have great potential.

Hospice / Step-down Facility

This twenty-two-bedded hospice / step-down facility would consist of two eight-bedder wards and a pediatric wards consisting of six beds. We will concentrate mainly on providing nursing care for the patients with doctors available on call. This is a step-down facility as well as a hospice, and we will not only care for terminally ill patients. Chronically ill patients who no longer require active medical care in hospital, but who are still not well enough to receive only part time home care will also benefit greatly from this facility. Once patients are well enough to go home, they can then be referred to our home-based caregivers. It is hoped that this facility will be up and running during the course of 2003.

However even though the local State Government are willing to pay for the running costs of this place of chronic care / hospice, they can not give any money towards capital costs, as it will be built on our land. Law prevents government from providing capital for buildings on privately owned land. This cost of building this facility is about $200,000 and currently this is all that stands between us and fulfilling the incredible God-given opportunities we have.

We feel that God has set us up for such a time as this. Never before has such a great opportunity been afforded to the church, and we must have the courage of our faith to attempt to great things for God.

How can Churches / Christians in America get involved or help out?

By sending short term mission teams:

These teams could be: Practically orientated in terms of building/maintenance, Sport evangelism teams, Holiday Bible club/children's work teams, Medical missionaries who would stay between one to two years (this requires pre-registration with the South African Medical and Dental Council), General Administrative helpers.

Funding

There are various funding opportunities for ongoing running expenses, staff salaries and capital projects. Details of these can be provided if needed.

Contact Details:

Living Hope Community Center
Pastor John V. Thomas
P O Box 1700
Sun Valley 7985
Tel: + 27(0) 21 785 4200
Facsimile: + 27(0) 21 785 3586
E-mail: john@livinghope.co.za
www.livinghope.co.za

African Leadership
P.O. Box 682444
Franklin, TN 37068-2444
E-mail: info@africanleadership.org

Prepared by Wendy Reedamd John Thomas, Living Hope Community Center

HOW TO PROVIDE MEALS FOR HOMELESS CHILDREN

Joan, a young woman famous among the street children of Harari, offers tea and bread as a substantial daily meal. She needs to raise support for uniforms, books, tuition costs, and living expenses for children who otherwise would be abandoned to the streets. Rev. and Mrs. David Kidd of Nashville, Tennessee decided to support this cause, and here's how they did it:

1. We visited Zimbabwe and God "rubbed our noses" in this awful need.
2. David did a sermon asking for donors from the congregation (in the form of modest monthly pledges).
3. We began with pledges of about $350 per month, with our benevolence team promising to match this money with benevolence money from the church coffers.
4. We set up our team (comprised of people who had visited Zimbabwe) and began communicating on a monthly basis with our donors. Sometimes we send little gifts such as doilies which have been crocheted by the ladies in Joan's sewing project.
5. The word spread: A member took a videotape to her parents' church in FL (a church that doesn't do much outreach) and some people there became monthly donors.

Also, a couple in Connecticut, got in touch with us and became very substantial donors, putting us over the top in our dream to buy a permanent residence for the ministry.

6. Recently, the Outreach Foundation of the Presbyterian Church recognized our project as a good cause and offered to "back up" our funding if it ever depleted. This is a great resource and contact because it takes the pressure off of us as individuals.

People will always respond to human suffering if you offer them a "convenient" way to help. The process is pretty much three fold:

1. Tell the story to the congregation

2. Offer them a concrete way to help

3. Keep in touch by articulating how their contribution is helping . . . so that the reality of what they are doing lives in their minds so that they stay committed to the cause. For example see our August donor letter:

Dear Friends,

As we suffer through the heat of another summer, winter has come to Zimbabwe.

I close my eyes and imagine the street children huddling down in their favorite sleeping places, snuggling in the comfort of the blankets which your dollars have provided. I think of them gathering in the early morning, waiting for Joan, their "Tea and Bread Lady" to arrive, her car filled with huge pots of hot, sweet tea, bread and peanut butter which your dollars have purchased. I smile, realizing that now, close to one hundred of those same children are attending school, thanks to your generosity.

Conditions in Zimbabwe grow worse by the season: a corrupt government, a depreciating currency, terrible food shortages, the growing AIDS crisis, all make life more difficult than ever for the street children. And yet, because of (name of church / organization)'s commitment to the Tea and Bread Ministry, there's still good news to report.

Many women and young girls from the street come daily to Joan's Home of Hope for sewing lessons. They gather there surrounded by an assortment of children to learn marketable sewing skills, to sing, pray and to enjoy hot nourishing meals cooked by the Home of Hope staff.

The Home of Hope compound has undergone significant improvements. A garage has been converted into a home for a Kim and Lucy and their young child, a couple who would be on the street with out this facility. Lucy is a skilled teacher and helps Joan with her classes, shopping and meal preparation, while Kim serves as the maintenance man. A second out building has been made into a home for Wilson, an elderly man rescued from the streets who gardens and does odd jobs around the compound.

With food shortages come long lines and huge hassles. Because Joan has a good, reliable car and enough money to purchase the food needed to carry on her feeding programs (and most important of all, the prayers of so many of you), her needs are continually being met.

But, just in case bread becomes impossible to purchase, Joan is in the process of stocking baking trays and ready mix bread flour to bake the bread at the Home of Hope.

In early August, another school term ends and Joan will be busy checking on the children's progress, purchasing needed uniforms and arranging for enrollment for the next term. I'm sure we will have more news of the school children in our next communication.

God is certainly good to allow us this opportunity to be actively involved in bringing His love and care to the streets of Harare, Zimbabwe. Please remember to pray for His children there. And never forget this truth: those homeless children who sleep, even now, under the blankets which you, their American friends, have provided . . . these very precious children of God . . . pray daily for you.

With love,
(Name of Director)

Once the money is raised, it is deposited into a special fund which has been established as a part of our church Benevolence account. Because there are many problems regarding the transfer of money to such a third world country, we have hired a "middle man," a member of the Presbyterian Church in Zimbabwe.

We send the money to an account he has established for this purpose and he acts as a bookkeeper for the ministry, paying the workers, providing the money for school fees etc for the children we have in school, and covering all financial needs as they arise.

We maintain our funds by keeping the donors motivated. As indicated earlier, we do this by regular communication and through occasional "gifts" such as the crocheted doilies or other small objects from Zimbabwe. We stay current with our donors by requiring monthly activity reports from Joan and her crew and include this information in our monthly letters.

To make this kind of a project work, I believe it's important to begin with a small group of people who understand the ministry firsthand and are on the same page.

If you can locate a person associated with a particular organization (in our case, the Presbyterian church) who can plug you in to a particular need, great! But that's a lot easier said than done. Most organizations simply need dollars to do their thing. Most individuals are hungry for personal involvement. There's a great divide between these two camps.

When we travel to Zimbabwe, we each take the largest bags we can get by with and they are totally stuffed with medicines, toys, etc. for the street children. This is another way that we have managed to keep people involved personally in the project. We put out a "wish list," and church members purchase things for us to take. We come back with photos of the children receiving these gifts.

To develop a personal connection with the community, we connect with one person at a time. You can't stand back and connect. In our case we go out onto the streets and help Joan serve her tea and bread. We play with the children, hold the babies, and encourage the adults to tell us their stories. At night we walk the streets, delivering food and blankets to those who are cold and hungry. I think you just have to be willing to go and be with the people. We take lots of photos and bring them back to tell the stories.

I can wrap up my amazement in one visual image. It is an image which I often share with our donors:

> *Each morning when the first rays of sun break over the city of Harare, in a little country called Zimbabwe in the south of Africa a stream of homeless people begin to gather on a certain corner. Children come from back alleys and out of storm drains, and from underneath bushes in the park. Many carry younger siblings or shepherd fellow orphans who have come recently from rural villages to make their way on the city streets. They arrive with bottles and cans they have dug out of garbage bins to come and sit in the first light and wait for the lady who brings tea and bread.*
>
> *Finally, she arrives, with vats of steaming sweet tea to fill their containers, and bread, spread on a good day, with peanut butter. But then before tea is served or bread broken . . . something staggering happens. The children sit on the dirty curb and bow their heads. They pray, giving thanks for the bounty they are about to enjoy. They always end their prayers with this: ". . . and God, please bless the good people in America who give us this bread and tea."*
>
> *Yes, each day, the street children of Zimbabwe are praying for me, and for you, and for all the people who participate in this endeavor.*

There are no words to express the wonder of this truth.

To contact Joan, write to:
Hillsboro Presbyterian Church
5820 Hillsboro Rd
Nashville, TN 37215-4602
Phone (615) 665-0148
DKidd@edge.net

Or, your organization can support another "Joan" in a different city, to expand the work done in Africa.

Prepared by Pam Kidd.

EPILOGUE

The New Plague

Franklin Graham
President, Samaritan's Purse

Dear Reader,

When I was asked to include my chapter in The aWAKE Project, *I was pleased to do this because of the extreme urgency of the HIV/AIDS crisis in Africa. As an evangelist and humanitarian worker, I believe the answer for the HIV/AIDS crisis lies in obedience to God's standards. I know that other contributors to this book may not agree, but the one thing we all agree upon is that something must be done to save as many as we possibly can. I believe the only hope for individuals is to conform to God's standards and laws in strict obedience. My hope is that in reading my thoughts, you will be inspired and motivated to act on behalf of this struggling continent.*

Sincerely,
Franklin Graham

When Jesus encountered people who wanted His healing touch, He never questioned them about how they became sick.

The Bible says:

And Jesus went about all Galilee, teaching in their synagogues, preaching the gospel of the kingdom, and healing all kinds of sickness and all kinds of disease among the people . . . and they brought to Him all sick people who were afflicted with various diseases and torments, and those who were demon-possessed, epileptics, and paralytics; and He healed them.[1]

Jesus was not condemning nor condescending. Why is that? We have to remember His mission. He came for the sick, not the healthy. He came for sinners, not the righteous. This was His mission. "Those who are well have no need of a physician, but those who are sick. I did not come to call the righteous, but sinners, to repentance."[2]

Many times organizations and businesses lose sight of their mission statement. You would be surprised how many people today do not even know the mission statement of the organization where they work, or the ministry in which they are involved. Jesus always had a clear focus and His mission was ever before Him: "to call sinners to repentance"—a very good lesson for you and me.

He used many different methods of healing, but He never prescreened individuals or sent them away because of previous sins. He dealt with the truth of their sins with love and mercy. He did not have to ask questions. He searched hearts and knew that all needed forgiveness and His healing touch. He forgave the woman caught in the act of adultery, which we read in the Scripture:

Now early in the morning He came again into the temple, and all the people came to Him; and He sat down and taught them. Then the scribes and Pharisees brought to Him a woman caught in adultery. And when they had set her in the midst, they said to Him, "Teacher, this woman was caught in adultery, in the very act. Now Moses, in the law, commanded us that such should be stoned. But what do You say?" This they said, testing Him, that they might have something of which to accuse Him. But Jesus stooped down and wrote on the ground with His finger, as though He did not hear. So when they continued asking Him, He raised Himself up and said to them, "He who is without sin among you, let him throw a stone at her first." And again He stooped down and wrote on the ground. Then those who heard it, being convicted by their conscience, went out one by one, beginning with the oldest even to the last. And Jesus was left alone, and the woman standing in the midst. When Jesus had raised Himself up and saw no one but the woman, He said to her, "Woman, where are those accusers of yours? Has no one condemned you?" She said, "No one, Lord." And Jesus said to her, "Neither do I condemn you; go and sin no more."[3]

There is a pandemic of death and destruction loose in our world today that demands the same nonjudgmental response from those who serve others in the Name of Jesus. The pandemic that I speak of is Acquired Immunodeficiency Syndrome, or AIDS, which is caused by the HIV (Human Immunodeficiency Virus). Millions are sick and dying without knowledge of the Son of the living God and the healing power that comes through His Name. Tens of millions will become ill and die in the years to come. It is a plague like those visited upon Egypt during the days of Moses in the Jewish captivity. The World Health Organization has called it "the most devastating disease humankind has ever faced."[4] The virus that causes AIDS has no known cure, no preventive vaccine, nor any hope of successful

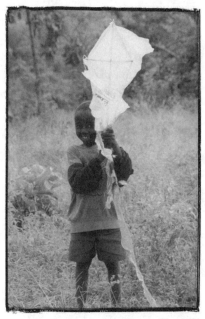

Courtesy of Pam Kidd

treatment in the near future. There are expensive drugs that can prolong life for a while, but for the most part, these can be afforded only by the wealthy. Still, they are not a cure.

When AIDS first came onto the world scene, many wanted to

stigmatize it as a homosexual problem, saying, "They are just getting what they deserve." For various reasons, most Christians-including myself-wanted to stay as far away from the issue as possible.

It is true that sinful behavior by homosexuals is a major factor in the spread of this deadly plague. But it is also true that in Africa, India, the Caribbean, and many other parts of the world, including the United States, HIV/AIDS is also caused by sinful heterosexual behavior, which threatens to annihilate men, women, and-sadly-children of an entire generation.

To many, Christians think of AIDS as a sinner's disease. No question, there are consequences to our actions, and we have to take responsibility for the choices we make in life.

As a pilot, if I fly at forty-one thousand feet and stick my head out the window of a pressurized airplane, I will not be able to survive more than just a few minutes, if that long. Why? Because I am outside the boundaries that God created for me to live a healthy life. I like to scuba dive (though I'm not very good at it). But if I stick my head just an inch under the water without a breathing apparatus, I will not last more than a few minutes, if that long. Why? Because I am outside the boundaries God created.

Likewise, when sex is experienced outside the boundaries God established-which is the marriage relationship between husband and wife-it threatens our health and even our very life. Why? Because we are engaging in behavior that is outside the boundaries God designed for us.

The church of Jesus Christ has a tremendous opportunity to reach out to those living with AIDS. Little has been said to those who are without hope of cure-those who are already infected and living with AIDS. Too often we have just looked the other way. I believe strongly that the way the church chooses to respond to HIV/AIDS, which is both a moral and a health crisis, will define how seriously our generation takes the Great Commission.

In past generations, Christians responded to the Great Commission by going to China to preach the Gospel, as my grandfather did. Other generations went to the jungles of Southeast Asia and Africa. Every generation seems to encounter some challenge that tests its resolve. Brave Christian servants like David Livingstone in Africa, and William Wilberforce in England, rallied the church to fight slavery and help break the chains of the oppressed. Over the next twenty years, one of the great mission fields for our generation will be to reach out to the 100 million people who will be infected with HIV and possibly die without ever hearing the Gospel of Jesus Christ.

This topic is difficult to discuss, which is why it is often ignored. But Jesus never shied away from tough issues. His ministry encompassed disagreement and conflicts. I believe that if He were physically present on earth today, He would be reaching out to those engulfed by this disease. He would show love and compassion, and would use His healing power in order to draw men, women, and children to Himself, even in the face of HIV/AIDS. Now throughout the world, millions are dying alone, rejected, hopeless-captives of a hideous sickness. Just how will we respond?

Background of a Crisis

When I first became aware of HIV/AIDS during the 1980s, I was appalled. The Bible pulls no punches in labeling sin. Sin is sin. God's response to wickedness is without prejudice. Every sinner, regardless of the sins committed, needs redemption found in the cross of Christ. Jesus came to save sinners, not to condemn them. The Bible says: "For God did not send His Son into the world to condemn the world, but that the world through Him might be saved."[5] Jesus ate with sinners, He talked with them, and He visited with them in their homes. This was one of the chief complaints of the religious leaders of that day. He associated with sinners; they did not. You see, Jesus' mission statement was always in clear focus.

Because of the ministry at Samaritan's Purse, my first real insight into understanding this pandemic was through missionary hospitals in other countries. Our ministry has watched this plague unfold before our eyes, primarily in Africa. Since the late 1970s, we have been sending doctors and nurses to clinics and hospitals in Africa.

When the disease which became known as AIDS was first identified in the early 1980s, we asked personnel in these missionary hospitals, "Have you seen any AIDS patients?" the answer was "No." But it wasn't long until reports trickled in that a few people were showing up as HIV-positive. Five years later, the number of hospital beds occupied by patients suffering with AIDS had increased to 10 to 20 percent of the hospital's total bed count. In some locations in Africa, 50 percent or more of the patients in hospitals now suffer with AIDS or AIDS-related diseases.

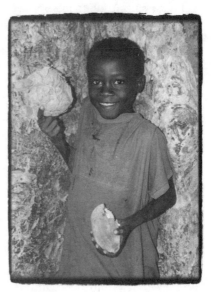

Courtesy of Pam Kidd

Unfortunately, when those sick with AIDS come to missionary hospitals there is little to do for them in terms of medicine because there is no cure, and no hope of a cure. We make them as comfortable as possible and help them die with dignity. In the process, we have the opportunity to point them to eternal life. Every person has a soul, and the greatest thing that we can do is to share with each and every one the hope that we have in Jesus Christ, the Savior of our souls.

Why is HIV/AIDS spreading so rapidly in third world nations?

The answer is a tangle of moral, social, physical, economic, and environmental factors. Of significant embarrassment to me is that American culture and mass media contribute to a sexually promiscuous mind-set that aggressively promotes alternative lifestyles that are against God's commands. I believe this has accelerated the spread of HIV.

For decades American TV and movies have been popular in other nations. The story lines in our entertainment have increasingly glorified sexual activity of all types outside of marriage. In most television entertainment, some type of extramarital sexual contact is suggested, endorsed, or depicted. Hollywood portrays fornication and adultery as attractive and glamorous. The people who do these things appear to get by without negative consequences; everyone looks happy, and physical lust reigns.

This scenario does not reflect reality, of course. Much of the world, however, looks up to America and the West because of material, political, scientific, and military achievements, and the freedoms we enjoy. They want to emulate the Western lifestyle that they have seen portrayed on television, where promiscuity is prevalent.

There are other causes, of course. In Africa, like so many other parts of the world, more jobs are available in the large cities. For many families in rural villages, a man must leave his wife and children and go far away to the city. Because of the cost and difficulty of transportation, he may be gone for many months or even years. While away, he may get involved with prostitutes—the city slums are full of brothels populated by impoverished women who have also fled to the city to survive. With few alternatives available, these women turn to one of the oldest trades in the world—that is, to sell themselves—often for pennies. It is an evil cycle that leads to despair and the proliferation of sin that can end in death.

The statistics on the HIV/AIDS crisis are alarming:

- In 2001, three million people died of AIDS.
- Worldwide AIDS is the fourth leading cause of death.[6]
- An estimated 28,000,000 people have already died of AIDS.[7] Of these, 70 percent lived in sub-Saharan Africa.[8] In this region there are more than 13.5 million AIDS orphans.[9]
- About thirteen million children have lost one or both parents to AIDS.
- In seven African countries, more than 20 percent of the 15-49 age-group is infected with HIV.[10]

- In the small African nation of Swaziland, 32 percent of the population is infected with HIV, and there are forty thousand AIDS orphans.[11]
- The majority of the AIDS patients in South Africa are ages 15-30.[12] Some communities in Africa have lost their entire population from age twenty through the mid-forties.
- Every 10 seconds, someone in the world is infected with the HIV virus,[13] and there are 5 million new HIV-infected persons each year. Worldwide, approximately 40 million people are infected with HIV (some say this a very conservative number).
- India and the Caribbean regions are now reporting the highest rates of increase in HIV infections.
- Every day 1,800 babies are born infected with HIV. Worldwide, 2.7 million children are infected. Each month, 50 thousand boys and girls die of AIDS.

Of the forty million people who are infected worldwide, many have become HIV-positive because of their own sinful behavior. Representing the greatest tragedy in this new plague are the innocent victims of this deadly disease who have become infected through the sinful behavior of others, often by loved ones who engaged in promiscuous sex, extramarital affairs, homosexual relationships, prostitution, or intravenous drug use, and then transmitted the virus to them. A small percentage have been infected through transfusions of contaminated blood or they were born HIV-positive because their mothers were infected.

In Western nations like the United States, those who are HIV positive have access to some medications that control or slow down the virus. But there is no cure or any hope for a successful vaccine in the foreseeable future. The question for Christians is the same as the question that appears on the popular WWJD bracelets worn today—"What Would Jesus Do?"

One thing I know for sure: He would not turn His back. Jesus would use His power as the Son of God to heal bodies, minds, and hearts.

So what can we do? With no cure for HIV/AIDS available, some type of alternative plan is needed because of the grim outlook. Here's a scenario built on valid assumptions: Some researchers report that a vaccine, which will be effective in offering protection against AIDS, may be ten or more years away. With the current rate at which the number of people infected with HIV is escalating, it is estimated that the number of people who are infected may reach fifty million over the next ten years. Added to the forty million who are already infected, that means close to one hundred million people will be HIV-positive by 2012! The estimated death toll for 2001, due to AIDS, was three million. That's three million lost lives. It is reasonable to assume the death toll will rise each year. Even assuming that no increase occurs, and present numbers stay the same, thirty million or more people can be expected to die of AIDS during the next decade. All are souls for whom Christ died and shed His blood on Calvary's cross.

We must do something on behalf of the Name.

A Battle Strategy

Although this virus and disease have no cure now, I do think the epidemic can be contained. It won't happen in one or two years, but through biblically based education, lifestyle changes, and certainly by proclaiming the Gospel, broken lives can be transformed and the tide turned.

In February of 2002, Samaritan's Purse hosted an international HIV/AIDS conference in Washington, D.C., called Prescription for Hope. Our ministry thought it was of absolute importance to assemble Christian workers who are on the front line in fighting this disease around the world. We also wanted to show how some in the church are already involved in this battle. But the role of the church needs to increase. So far, the homosexual community and the United Nations have had the loudest voices on the issue. The church has an unprecedented opportunity to take the love of Jesus Christ and the hope that is found in Him to millions who may never otherwise hear how God can change their lives. True, government agencies have not always invited the church to the table to share their views, but perhaps this can change as the church becomes more involved in reaching out to those who are facing this horrible epidemic. It's important to note, however, that in hospitals, clinics, and dispensaries around the world, Christian missionaries and national workers have quietly been on the forefront of treating HIV/AIDS victims, as well as aiding orphans and providing hospice care.

The conference convened with nearly one thousand in attendance from eighty-six countries, including physicians, missionary AIDS workers, church leaders, representatives of humanitarian foundations and compassionate care ministries, and government officials. About one-third of those present were "frontline" providers of care to HIV/AIDS patients.

As a result of this conference and our previous experience, I would like to suggest several components of a strategy that I believe needs to be mounted on behalf of the church in an effort to combat HIV/AIDS:

Leadership

The church should be leading, not following or watching this fight. Let's stop waiting for the government or the medical or scientific industry to solve this problem. Let's put this issue at the top of our agendas as individuals, churches, denominations, and Christian organizations.

A Time magazine cover story dated February 12, 2001, stated:

> Without treatment, those with HIV will sicken and die; without prevention, the spread of infection cannot be checked. South Africa has no other means available to break the vicious cycle except to change everyone's sexual behavior-and that is not happening. The essential missing ingredient is leadership. Neither the countries of the region nor those of the wealthy world have been able or willing to provide it.[14]

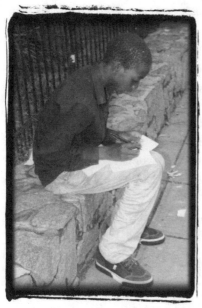
Courtesy of Pam Kidd

The church must help meet the leadership deficit not only in South Africa but also in the rest of the world.

The church must stop the finger-pointing and condemnation. "See, we told you so," is not going to cut it. This is about as effective as yelling "baby killers" at young girls going into abortion clinics. That will not change a girl's heart. But if we reach out in love and compassion to individuals with HIV/AIDS, we can try to win them to faith in Jesus Christ. Everyone needs forgiveness and cleansing from unrighteousness and the hope of eternal life in heaven.

Jesus came to rescue sinners. People infected with HIV/AIDS are sinners, the same as you and me.

Education

An education effort developed in Uganda has been a key in lowering the HIV infection rate from around 30 percent to less than 10 percent in that country. Their curriculum was developed by a missionary and was mandated by Uganda's president to be taught in every school. This Bible-based approach should be duplicated elsewhere.

Education requires telling the truth concerning improper sexual behavior and how HIV and other diseases can be transmitted through it. It is shocking to learn how many millions still do not know the most basic information about how HIV is transmitted and how it can be prevented. Knowledge is power. The more men and women know, the more control they will have over their lives. It does not necessarily mean that just because people "know," they will not engage in risky behavior; some people will continue to live questionable lifestyles in spite of all the warnings.

Men and women must be educated about the risk associated with lifestyles and behavior that are outside of God's boundaries. Pastors everywhere should include in their preaching and teaching sexual abstinence before marriage and faithfulness to one's husband or wife in marriage, as the Bible teaches: "Since there is so much immorality, each man should have his own wife, and each woman her own husband."[15]

As I have carefully read the literature concerning HIV/AIDS, it has become very obvious to me that condoms are not the answer. There are scientific reports that show condoms, if properly used, may offer some degree of protection against HIV and other sexually transmitted diseases, but distribution of condoms encourages promiscuous sexual behavior. For the last ten years, the United Nations and world health organizations, along with the United States government, have distributed hundreds of millions of condoms. In spite of this mass distribution, the HIV/AIDS infection rate has continued to climb. *The only answer for reversing the tide is to adopt God's standards for sexual behavior: abstinence before marriage and faithfulness to one's spouse, of the opposite sex, in marriage.*

Allocation of resources

Where possible, the church needs to work with governments and other agencies around the world to help them allocate resources to education and programs that are worthwhile. I am thankful that the United States government contributes one-third of the aid for the fight against HIV/AIDS worldwide.[16] It is only fitting that we do this since our declining moral values, found in our popular music, movies, and television programming, are a contributing cause to the spread of HIV.

Present Clearly the Hope That We Have in Jesus Christ

I am not naive about human nature. HIV/AIDS is getting a great deal of attention because there is no cure and it leads to certain death, but there are a number of other sexually transmitted diseases. Some have no cure. Some can be treated, but researchers report that resistance to current medications is occurring. All sexually transmitted diseases can lead to pain and suffering. These can devastate health and, in some instances, cause death. No matter how much we educate, sin will still deceive, and people will still engage in life-threatening, high-risk behavior to get a moment of sexual gratification. But isn't it possible to make a dent? If we can reduce the annual infection rate by just 20 percent through biblically based education, that would prevent the infection of one million people each year, or 40 percent-two million people-all souls of utmost importance to God. There is not a cure for HIV/AIDS. But there is hope if we turn to God and follow His laws and commands. This battle can be won in time and with His help. It can be done.

Followers of Jesus Christ should reach out in love to those who do not have the same hope that we have in Christ Jesus. "Love suffers long and is kind . . . bears all things, believes all things, hopes all things, endures all things. Love never fails."[17] Let's reach out in ways in which we have never reached out before and demonstrate with actions-and not just words-that we care for others because God cares. Every soul is precious in the sight of God. Shouldn't every soul be precious in our sight?

The Call to Battle

My desire is to see an army of Christian men and women going out across the globe to wage war against HIV/AIDS. Ultimately, every army is only as strong as its soldiers. The army of the Lord Jesus Christ is no different. I want to tell just one story of an individual "foot soldier" in the war against HIV/AIDS.

I first met this Canadian ball of energy, Avis Rideout, at the Prescription for Hope conference. Avis has a passion to see both babies with AIDS and sinners find new life.

When Avis and her husband, Roy, went to Thailand as missionaries in 1972, neither of them ever imagined they would someday be frontline soldiers, battling a horrible disease. Avis was a nurse, but at that time HIV/AIDS had not even appeared as a health issue. Thailand, long known for its sexual promiscuity, soon became one of Asia's most infected countries.

In the mid-1990s Avis's understanding of God's intentions for her life were radically altered during a visit to a government-sponsored hospital ward for babies who were HIV-positive. While there, Avis saw babies, sick and dying because of the actions of others, lying on their mats, some with swollen stomachs and covered with sores-all untouched and alone. Because of fear, believing that even the slightest contact with the sick infants might put them at risk of contracting HIV, caregivers wore rubber gloves and kept as far away as they could from these tiny ones who had no one to love them.

"I saw that these babies were dying, not from HIV, but from rejection," Avis says. Her heart broke.

She and Roy saw a baby girl named Nikki. She had lost her hair and was "skin and bones" and about to die. Moved by the compassion of Christ, they decided to take her home. Not long after, the Rideouts opened the Agape Home, a place devoted solely to the care of HIV infants.

Since then, 129 HIV babies have arrived at Agape Home where each one is held, touched, kissed, and loved. Avis says, "It's about giving quality life, and hope when there is no hope. We have seen fantastic results, because we are able to bring them in and love and care for them . . . through touching, holding, and talking to them."

Each child receives medical and nutritional care. But best of all each one is given a tender, personal touch and love in the Name of Jesus. And no child ever dies alone. Members of the staff hold the dying infant, expressing affection softly, and singing of the love of Jesus, repeating verses of comfort from Scripture. Some of these children, like Nikki, have grown and are strong. Many would appear to be normal children. In Nikki's case, she is still HIV-positive. Someday she will die, but if it were not for Avis and Roy, Nikki and 129 others would have been discarded with no hope. Each child that comes into this home is given something he or she desperately needs, and that is love: the love of Christ that flows through those who carry His Name. Jesus says, "Inasmuch as you did it to one of the least of these My brethren, you did it to me."[18]

At the Prescription for Hope conference, Avis made clear that there is a disease more deadly than AIDS. "I am an evangelist," she said. "My heart throbs constantly for the lost souls of this world. I see in America, and other countries around the world, a greater disease than AIDS-it is sin . . . Sin is death. But there is eternal hope and peace through Jesus Christ . . . If there had been just one AIDS baby dying without hope, God would have sent His Son to save that one child."

Avis is so right. By ministering to the millions—young and old— we can go on a rescue mission to save those infected with AIDS and those blinded by sin by sharing with them God's grace, mercy, and forgiveness found only through the Name.

Reprinted by permission of Franklin Graham.
From The Name, *Copyright © 2002 by Thomas Nelson Publishers.*

NOTES

Rachel Gbenyon-Diggs

1. Declaration of Commitment, United Nations Special Session on HIV/AIDS, 25-27 June, 2001, NY/A/RES/S-26, Para2.

2. The New Partnership for Africa's Development (NEPAD), October 2001, p.37, Para 125.

3. The World Bank, World Development Report, 1985, (Oxford University Press, 1986), passim.

4. J. Gus Liebenow, LIBERIA, The Quest for Democracy, (Indiana University Press, 1987), p.1.

5. John W. Gardner, Excellence, Can We Be Equal And Excellent Too?, (W.W. Norton, New York, London), 1961.

6. Ibid.

7. Ibid.

Helen Epstein and Lincoln Chen

1. See *George Soros on Globalization* (Public Affairs, 2002).

2. See *AIDS in the World*, edited by Jonathan Mann, Daniel Tarantola, and Thomas Netter (Harvard University Press, 1992) and references therein.

3. See "Viagra Is a $50 Million Pentagon Budget Item," *The New York Times*, October 4, 1998. The actual amount spent on Viagra turned out to be far less than this, however. 4. See Helen Epstein's article "The Mystery of AIDS in South Africa," *The New York Review*, July 20, 2000.

4. In addition, the US contribution will not consist of entirely new funds, but will be largely taken from existing international health programs, including those for maternal and child health in developing countries.

5. Paul Farmer and others, "Community-Based Approaches to HIV Treatment in Resource-Poor Settings," *The Lancet*, Vol. 358 (August 4, 2001).

NOTES

Richard Stearns

1. Luke 10:25, New King James Version
2. Luke 10:26, New King James Version
3. Luke 10:27, New King James Version
4. Luke 10:28, New King James Version
5. Luke 10: 29, New King James Version
6. Singer, Peter. *Practical Ethics.* Cambridge: Cambridge University Press, 1993.
7. "Americans' Interest in Assisting the International AIDS Crisis," National survey of U.S. Adults conducted by Barna Research Group, Ltd., Ventura, CA, January 2001.
8. Dr. Gary Gulbranson, Senior Pastor, Westminster Chapel, Bellevue, WA.
9. James 1:22, New King James Version
10. James 2: 14-17, New King James Version
11. Luke 10:36, New King James Version
12. Luke 10:37, New King James Version
13. Luke 25:34-40, New King James Version
14. "What's So Amazing About Grace?" by Phillip Yancey. Copyright 1997 by Phillip Yancey.
15. Luke 10:37, New King James Version

Vladimir Bertaud, M.D.

1. UNAIDS/WHO. *AIDS epidemic update: December* 2000. Geneva, Joint United Nations Programme on HIV/AIDS and World Health Organization, 2000.
2. UNAIDS/WHO. *AIDS epidemic update: December* 2001. Geneva, Joint United Nations Programme on HIV/AIDS and World Health Organization 2001.
3. Gregson S, Nyamukapa CA, Garnett GP, et al. Sexual mixing patterns and sex-differentials in teenage exposure to HIV infection in rural Zimbabwe. *The Lancet* 2002; 359: 1896-1903.
4. Kaleebu P, French N, Mahe C, et al. Effect of Human Immunodeficiency Virus (HIV) type 1 envelope subtypes A and D on disease progression in a large cohort of HIV-1 positive persons in Uganda. *J Infect Dis* 2002; 185 (9): 1244-50.
5. Loemba H, Brenner B, Parniak MA, et al. Genetic Divergence of Human Immunodeficiency Virus Type 1 Ethiopian Clade C Reverse Transcriptase (RT) and Rapid Development of resistance against nonnucleoside inhibitors of RT. *Antimicrob Agents Chemother* 2000; 46 (7): 2087-94.
6. Morgan D, Mahe C, Mayanja B, Whitworth JAG. Progression to symptomatic disease in people infected with HIV-1 in rural Uganda: prospective cohort study. *BMJ* 2002; 324: 193-197.
7. Salamon R, Marimoutou C, Ekra D, et al. *J Acquir Immune Defic Syndr* 2002; 29 (2): 149-57.

8. Morgan D, Mahe C, Mayanja B, Okongo JM, Lubega R, Whitworth JA. *AIDS* 2002; 16 (4): 597-603.

9. Colebunders R, Francis H, Mann JM, et al. Persistent diarrhea, strongly associated with HIV infection in Kinshasa, Zaïre. *Am J Gastroenterol* 1987; 82: 859-864.

10. Sewankambo N, Mugerwa RD, Goodgame RW, *et al.* Enteropathic AIDS in Uganda: an endoscopic, histological and microbiological study. *AIDS* 1987; 1: 9-13.

11. Colebunders R, Mann JM, Francis H, et al. Generalized papular pruritic eruption in African patients with human immunodeficiency virus infection. *AIDS* 1987; 1: 117-121.

12. Tyndall MW, Nasio J, Agoki E, et al. Herpes Zoster as the initial presentation of human immunodeficiency virus type 1 infection in Kenya. *Clin Infect Dis* 1995; 21: 1035-7.

13. Graham SM, Daley HM, Ngwira B. Finger clubbing and HIV infection in Malawian children. *Lancet* 1997; 349: 31.

14. Reeve PA, Harries AD, Nkhoma WA, et al. Clubbing in African patients with pulmonary tuberculosis. *Thorax* 1987; 42: 986-87.

15. Gilks CF, Brindle RJ, Otieno LS, et al. Life-threatening bactaeremia in HIV-1 seropositive adults admitted to hospital in Nairobi, Kenya. *Lancet* 1990; 336: 545-9.

16. Gilks CF, Ojoo SA, Ojoo JC, et al. Invasive pneumococcal disease in a cohort of predominantly HIV-1 infected female sex-workers in Nairobi, Kenya. *Lancet* 1996; 347: 718-23.

17. Daley CL, Mugusi F, Chen LL, et al. Pulmonary complications of HIV infection in Dar es Salaam, Tanzania. *Am J Respir Crit Care Med* 1996; 154: 106-10.

18. Batungwanayo J, Taelman H, Lucas S, et al. Pulmonary disease associated with the human immunodeficiency virus in Kigali, Rwanda. *Am J Respir Crit Care Med* 1994; 149: 1591-6.

19. Malin AS, Gwanzura LZ, Klein S, et al. *Pneumocystis carinii* pneumonia in Zimbabwe. *Lancet* 1995; 346:1258-61.

20. De Cock KM, Gnaore E, Adjorlolo G, et al. Risk of tuberculosis in patients with HIV-1 and HIV-II infections in Abidjan, Ivory Coast. *BMJ* 1991; 302: 496-499.

21. Allen S, Batungwanayo J, Kerlikowske K, et al. Two-year incidence of tuberculosis in cohorts of HIV-infected and uninfected urban Rwandan women. Am Rev Respir Dis 1992; 146: 1439-1444.

22. De Cock KM, Soro B, Coulibaly IM, Lucas SB. Tuberculosis and HIV infection in sub-Saharan Africa. *JAMA* 1992; 268: 1581-1587.

23. Elliott AM, Luo N, Tembo G, et al. Impact of HIV on tuberculosis in Zambia: a cross sectional study. *BMJ* 1990; 301: 412-5.

24. Eriki PP, Okwera A, Aisu T, et al. The influence of human immunodeficiency virus infection on tuberculosis in Kampala, Uganda. *Am Rev Respir Dis 1991*; 143: 185-187.

25. Batungwanayo J, Taelman H, Dhote R, et al. Pulmonary tuberculosis in Kigali, Rwanda. Impact of human immunodeficiency virus infection on clinical and radiographic presentation. *Am Rev Respir Dis* 1992; 146: 53-56.

26. Harries AD. Tuberculosis and human immunodeficiency virus infection in developing countries. *Lancet* 1990; 335: 387-390.

27. Richter C, Perenboom R, Mtoni I, et al. Clinical features of HIV-seropositive and HIV-seronegative patients with tuberculous pleural effusion in Dar es Salaam, Tanzania. *Chest* 1994; 106: 1471-76.

28. Mukadi Y, Perriëns JH, St Louis ME, et al. Spectrum of immunodeficiency in HIV-1-infected patients with pulmonary tuberculosis in Zaire. *Lancet* 1993; 342: 143-146.

29. Ackah AN, Coulibaly D, Digbeu H, et al. Response to treatment, mortality, and CD4 lymphocyte counts in HIV-infected persons with tuberculosis in Abidjan, Côte d'Ivoire. *Lancet* 1995; 345: 607-610.

30. Maartens G, Willcox PA, Benatar S. Miliary tuberculosis: rapid diagnosis, hematologic abnormalities, and outcome in 109 treated adults. *Am J Med* 1990; 89: 291-296.

31. Archibald LK, den Dulk MO, Pallangyo KJ, and Reller LB. Fatal *Mycobacterium tuberculosis* bloodstream infections in febrile hospitalized adults in Dar es Slaam, Tanzania. *Clin Infect Dis* 1998; 26: 290-6.

32. Perriëns JH, Colebunders RL, Karahunga C, et al. Increased and tuberculosis treatment failure rate among human immunodeficiency virus (HIV) seropositive compared with HIV seronegative patients with pulmonary tuberculosis treated with "standard" chemotherapy in Kinshasa, Zaire. *Am Rev Resp Dis* 1991; 144: 750-755.

33. Elliott AM, Halwiindi B, Hayes RJ, et al. The impact of human immunodeficiency virus on response to treatment and recurrence rate in patients treated for tuberculosis: two-year follow-up of a cohort in Lusaka, Zambia. *J Trop Med Hyg* 1995; 98: 9-21.

34. Perriëns JH, St Louis ME, Mukadi YB, et al. Pulmonary tuberculosi in HIV-infected patients in Zaire. A controlled trial of treatment for either 6 or 12 months. *N Engl J Med* 1995; 332 (12): 779-784.

35. Davies GR, Connolly C, Wim Sturm A, et al. Twice-weekly, directly observed treatment for HIV-infected and uninfected tuberculosis patients: cohort study in rural South Africa. *AIDS* 1999; 13: 811-817.

36. Grosskurth H, Mosha F, Todd J, et al. Impact of improved treatment of sexually transmitted diseases on HIV infection in rural Tanzania: randomized controlled trial. *Lancet* 1995; 346: 530-36.

37. Wawer MJ, Sewankambo NK, Serwadda D et al. Control of sexually transmitted diseases for AIDS prevention in Uganda: a randomized community trial. *Lancet* 1999; 353: 525-35.

38. Hudson CP. AIDS in rural Africa: a paradigm for HIV-1 prevention. *AIDS* 1996; 7: 236-243.

39. Watts DH. Management of human immunodeficiency virus infection in pregnancy. *N Engl J Med* 2002; 346 (24): 1979-90.

40. Dorenbaum A. Report of results of PACTG 316: an international phase III trial of standard antiretroviral (ARV) prophylaxis plus nevirapine (NVP) for prevention of perinatal HIV transmission. In: Proceedings of the Eighth Conference on Retroviruses and Opportunistic Infections, Chicago, February 4-8, 2001: 277. Abstract.

41. Cooper ER, Charurat M, Mofenson L, et al. Combination antiretroviral strategies for the treatment of pregnant HIV-1 infected women and prevention of perinatal HIV-1 transmission. *J Acquir Immune Defic Syndr* 2002; 29: 484-94.

42. Scheduled cesarean delivery and the prevention of vertical transmission of HIV infection. No. 234. Washington, D.C.: American College of Obstetricians and Gynecologists, May 2000.

43. Wade NA, Birkhead GS, Warren BL, et al. Abbreviated regimens of zidovudine prophylaxis and perinatal transmission of the human immunodeficiency virus. *N Engl J Med 1998*; 339: 1409-14.

44. *MMWR* 1998; 47.

45. *MMWR 2000;* 49.

46. Wiktor SZ, Sassan-Morokro, Grant AD et al. Efficacy of trimethoprim-sulphamethoxazole prophylaxis to decrease morbidity and mortality in HIV-1 infected patients with tuberculosis in Abidjan, Côte d'Ivoire: a randomized controlled trial. *Lancet* 1999; 353: 1469-75.

47. Anglaret X, Chêne G, Attia A et al. Early chemoprophylaxis with trimethoprim-sulphamethoxazole for HIV-1 infected adults in Abidjan, Côte d'Ivoire: a randomized trial. *Lancet* 1999; 353: 1463-68.

48. Kelly P, Lungu F, Keane E et al. Albendazole chemotherapy for treatment of diarrhoea in patients with AIDS in Zambia: a randomized double blind controlled trial. *BMJ* 1996; 312: 1187-91.

49. Guinness L, Arthur G, Bhatt SM et al. Costs of hospital care for HIV-positive and HIV-negative patients at Kenyatta National Hospital, Nairobi, Kenya. *AIDS* 2002; 16 (6): 901-8.

50. Badri M, Wilson D, Wood R. Effect of highly active antiretroviral therapy on incidence of tuberculosis in South Africa: a cohort study. *Lancet* 2002; 359: 2059-64.

51. Weidle PJ, Malamba S, Mwebaze R et al. Assessment of a pilot antiretroviral drug therapy programme in Uganda: patients' response, survival, and drug resistance. *Lancet* 2002; 360: 34-40.

52. Mbulaiteye SM, Mahe C, Whitworth JAG et al. Declining HIV-1 incidence and associated prevalence over 10 years in a rural population in south-west Uganda: a cohort study. *Lancet* 2002; 360: 41-46.

53. Schultz AM, Bradac JA. The HIV vaccine pipeline, from preclinical to phase III. *AIDS* 2001; 15 (suppl 5): S147-58.

54. A Focus on Women. Third International Conference on Global Strategies for the Prevention of HIV Transmission from Mothers to Infants, Kampala, Uganda, September 9-13, 2001.

NOTES

John Waliggo

1. Cf. *Gaudium et Spes*, nos. 5 and 58, *Ad Gentes*, no. 22.

2. Monica K. Hellwig, *Jesus: The Compassion of God* (Dublin, 1983), p. 21.

3. Liberation theologians like Jon Sobrino have made an important distinction between "imitating" Jesus and "following" Jesus. The latter, as Sobrino explains, "is discipleship and takes into account the differences in Jesus' own time and out rime." *Christology at the Crossroads* (Maryknoll, N.Y.: Orbis Books, 1978), p. 389.

4. The author distributed questionnaires to 130 theological students of Gaba National Seminary, Uganda, with 66 responses. Some responses are discussed later in this paper.

5. Hellwig, p. 26.

6. The present experience of war in the Sudan between the Northern Arabic Muslims and the Southern black Christians and traditionalists is a precise example of this.

7. Sobrino, p. xv.

8. Ibid.

9. Ibid., p. xvi.

10. Andrew M. Greeley, *The Jesus Myth* (New York, 1973), p. 18.

11. Ibid., p. 31.

12. Ibid., p. 188.

13. Cf. *Populorum Progressio*, no 31.

14. Cf. Ecclesiastes 3:1-8.

15. P. D. Curtin, *The Atlantic Slave Trade: A Census* (Madison, 1967).

16. E. A. Bret, *Colonialism and Underdevelopment in East Africa* (London 1973 [sic]), L.H. Gann and P. Guignan (eds.), *Colonialism in Africa* (Cambridge, 1970).

17. UNCTAD Secretariat, *The History of UNCTAD 1964-1984* (New York, 1985).

18. *The Debt Crisis Network, From Debt to Development* (Washington, D.C., 1986).

19. Yoweeri K. Museveni, "The historical task of development," a paper presented to the 4th National Theological Week, Katigondo, 9th January 1989.

20. Cf. D. Martin, *General Amin* (London, 1974); A. Mazrui, *Soldiers and Kinsmen in Uganda*, London, 1975 [sic]; S.P. Panter-Brick (ed.), *Nigerian Politics and Military Rule* (London, 1970).

21. Adebayo Adedeji, *Can Our World Excape the Path of Mutual Injury and Self-destruction?* (Geneva, 1986).

22. Cf. Pope Nicholas V's Breif of 1452 to King Alfonso V of Portugal.

23. J. B. Webster, *African Churches in Yorubaland, 1888-1922* (london, 1964).

24. Cf. Jordan Winthrop, *White Over Black* (Baltimore, Maryland, 1969).

25. *Newsweek*, 20 February 1989, pp. 40-41.

26. Response no. 36 to the questionnaire.

NOTES

Franklin Graham

1. Matthew 4:23-24 NKJV.
2. Mark 2:17 NKJV.
3. John 8:2-11 NKJV.
4. "AIDS Epidemic Update—December 2001, Global Overview," Joint United Nations Programme on HIV/AIDS, 1. Accessed on the Internet at www.unaids.org, June 6, 2002.
5. John 3:17 NKJV.
6. Amy Fagan, "Christians Urged to Act Against HIV," *Washington Times*, 19 February 2002.
7. Raju Chebium, "N.C. Doctor Finds His Faith Helps on AIDS Mission," Gannett News Service, 21 February 2002.
8. Uwe Siemon-Netto, "Evangelicals to Ponder AIDS Pandemic," UPI, 9 November 2001.
9. Sheler, "Prescription for Hope."
10. Sharon Begley, "AIDS at 20," *Newsweek*, 11 June 2001, 36.
11. Carlyle Murphy, "'Army' of Christians Needed in AIDS Fight, Evangelist Says," *Washington Post*, 19 February 2002, B4.
12. Siemon-Netto, "Evangelicals to Ponder."
13. Uwe Soimon-Netto [sic], "Slow Church Response to AIDS Scolded," UPI, 18 February 2002.
14. Johanna McGeary, "Death Stalks a Continent," *Time* magazine, 12 February 2001. Accessed on the Internet at www.Time.com on 5 June 2002.
15. 1 Corinthians 7:2 NIV.
16. Murphy, "'Army' of Christians Needed in AIDS Fight, Evangelist Says," B1.
17. 1 Corinthians 13:4, 7-8 NKJV.
18. Matthew 25:40 NKJV.

DONATIONS

All contributors to The aWAKE Project *have waived their royalties. They are being donated to the following organizations:*

World Vision's Hope Initiative

The Hope Initiative is World Vision's global response to reduce the world-wide impact of HIV/AIDS. Introduced in October 2000 and officially launched in March 2001 with the appointment of Ken Casey to head the initiative, the Hope Initiative will expand and enhance World Vision's HIV/AIDS programming in all of the countries where it works.

The overall goal of the HIV/AIDS Hope Initiative is to reduce the global impact of HIV/AIDS through the enhancement and expansion of World Vision programs and collaborations focused on HIV/AIDS prevention, care, and advocacy.

Prevention: Making a significant contribution to the reduction of national HIV/AIDS incidence rates

Care: Achieving measurable improvement in the quality of life of children affected by HIV/AIDS

Advocacy: Encouraging the adoption of public policy and programs that will minimise the spread of HIV/AIDS and provide maximum care for those living with or affected by HIV/AIDS.

http://www.worldvision.org

Jubilee USA Network

Jubilee USA Network began as Jubilee 2000/USA in 1997 when a diverse gathering of people and organizations came together in response to the international call for Jubilee debt cancellation. Now over sixty organizations including labor, churches, religious communities and institutions, AIDS activists, trade campaigners and over nine thousand individuals are active members of the Jubilee USA Network. Together we are a strong, diverse and growing network dedicated to working for a world free of debt for billions of people.

In the Jubilee Year as quoted in Leviticus, those enslaved because of debts are freed, lands lost because of debt are returned, and community torn by inequality is restored. Today international debt has become a new form of slavery. Debt slavery means poor people working harder and harder in a vain effort to keep up with the interest payments on debts owed to rich countries including the U.S. and international financial institutions such as the International Monetary Fund (IMF) and the World Bank. Jubilee USA Network brings together people to turn this reality around by active solidarity with partners worldwide, targeted and timely advocacy strategies and educational outreach. Please join us in working for Jubilee justice.

http://www.j2000usa.org

ABOUT THE BOOK

The *aWAKE Project* is a unique and provocative book regarding the AIDS crisis in Africa. In June of 2001, Dr. Volney P. Gay, Chair of the Department of Religious Studies at Vanderbilt University, using a grant from the Templeton Foundation, conceived of a conference called *AIDS and Africa: Science and Religion* to take place on October 19, 2002. In June of 2002, he and Jenny Eaton, a Vanderbilt Ph.D. candidate and editor at Thomas Nelson, Inc., hosted a luncheon with Thomas Nelson colleagues David Moberg, Jerry Park, and Kate Etue. At that table was born *The aWAKE Project.*

The Vanderbilt conference unites persons across religious, political, and racial lines; this book embraces a spectrum of religious and political thought. The conference and this book help us confront ourselves and our responses to the AIDS pandemic.

The aWAKE Project was unveiled at the Vanderbilt University Conference on October 19, 2002.